# WEIGHTS on the
# BOSU®
# Balance Trainer

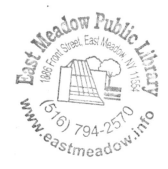

# WEIGHTS on the BOSU® Balance Trainer

## Strengthen and Tone All Your Muscles with Unstable Workouts

**Brett Stewart and Jason Warner**

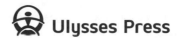 Ulysses Press

Published in the United States by
Ulysses Press
P.O. Box 3440
Berkeley, CA 94703
www.ulyssespress.com

ISBN13: 978-1-61243-127-7
Library of Congress Control Number 2012951895

Printed in the United States by Bang Printing

10 9 8 7 6 5 4 3 2 1

Acquisitions Editor: Keith Riegert
Managing Editor: Claire Chun
Editor: Lily Chou
Proofreader: Lauren Harrison
Index: Sayre Van Young
Front cover design: what!design @ whatweb.com
Interior design and production: Jake Flaherty
Interior photographs: © Scott E. Whitney except pages 107–10 and 112–15 © Rapt Productions
Front cover photographs: man © Eliza Snow/istockphoto.com; woman © Anthony Mayatt/istockphoto.com
Back cover photograph: © Scott E. Whitney
Models: Brian Burns, Tricia Burns, Lewis Elliot, Mary Gines, Brett Stewart, Kristen Stewart

BOSU® is a registered trademark of BOSU Fitness, LLC, and is protected under United States and international laws and is used under license from BOSU Fitness, LLC. The views expressed in this book are not endorsed by BOSU Fitness, LLC, and the author(s) of this book are in no way affiliated with, or sponsored by, BOSU Fitness, LLC.

Please Note

This book has been written and published strictly for informational purposes, and in no way should be used as a substitute for consultation with health care professionals. You should not consider educational material herein to be the practice of medicine or to replace consultation with a physician or other medical practitioner. The authors and publisher are providing you with information in this work so that you can have the knowledge and can choose, at your own risk, to act on that knowledge. The authors and publisher also urge all readers to be aware of their health status and to consult health care professionals before beginning any health program. This book is independently authored and published and no sponsorship or endorsement of this book by, and no affiliation with, any trademarked events, brands or other products mentioned or pictured within is claimed or suggested. All trademarks that appear in this book belong to their respective owners and are used here for informational purposes only. The authors and publisher encourage readers to patronize the quality events, brands and other products mentioned and pictured in this book.

*To our amazing wives, Kristen and Anne Marie. You've proven to us time and time again that you're incredibly adept at the most demanding balancing "workout" ever—being spectacular, selfless mothers.*

# Contents

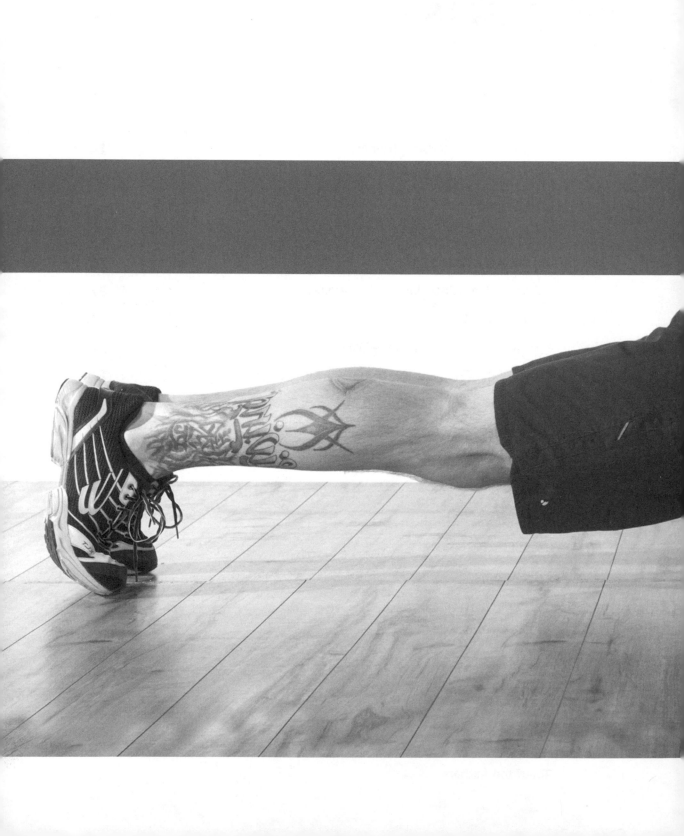

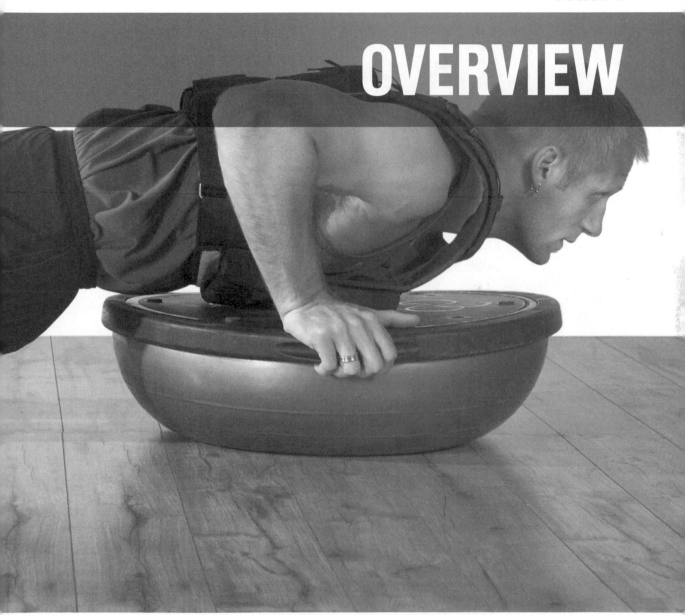

# Introduction

If you've set foot in nearly any gym, toning studio or rehab facility, then undoubtedly you've seen a BOSU Balance Trainer, its bulbous, blue, malleable dome beckoning you to hop on and test your balance while the solid black platform allays any fears of it being too unstable to support your weight. At first glance a BOSU Balance Trainer conveys everything you'll come to learn as fact in this book: Although completely unassuming, this cute-as-a-button marvel of simple technology all at once delivers a core-blasting, muscle-quivering challenge capable of working every muscle in your body to develop strength, agility and a toned physique.

Over the last decade, BOSU Balance Trainers have seemingly become one of the most successful pieces of exercise equipment sold worldwide and they can be found in more gyms across the globe than any other single brand of exercise equipment that doesn't contain a weight. The BOSU Balance Trainer is one of a kind in form and in function: The blue half-dome resembles a stability ball that has been split in half and secured to a black plastic serving tray, yet it's revered as the training tool of choice to develop core strength, stability and flexibility by athletes all over the world. As a go-to tool for trainers and physical therapists seeking to help their clients work their full body in many planes and stretch and strengthen major and supporting muscles, the BOSU Balance Trainer is unmatched in success and popularity.

Pairing weights with the unstable surface of the BOSU Balance Trainer reinforces the beneficial nature of lifting, twisting, pulling and pushing weights through an enhanced range of motion on multiple planes. By utilizing a BOSU Balance Trainer, the recruitment of supporting and stabilizing muscles is magnified to deliver a higher metabolic effect as well as boost muscle growth through time under tension on a non-uniform surface. Quite simply, you'll work more muscles more quickly while performing easy, repeatable weighted movements. By recruiting more muscles for stabilization, you'll also increase your metabolic rate and burn fat more quickly than just lifting weights alone!

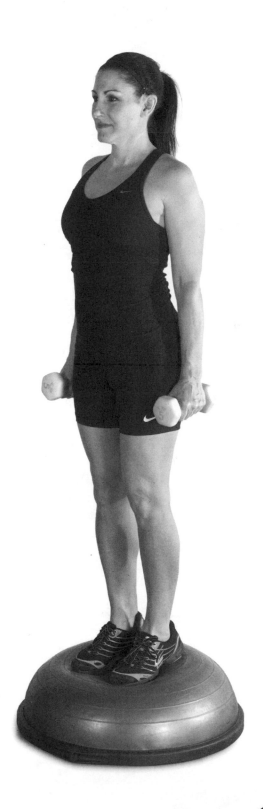

# About the Book

Who should read this book? Women. Men. Athletes. People recovering from injuries. People with too little time to get to the gym. People looking for a no-fuss, no-muss workout they can do with very little equipment in their living room. Really, anyone looking to improve their life and overall fitness level.

The BOSU Balance Trainer is an extraordinary device that allows a wide range of exercises. Combined with weights, it'll take your fitness and body to whole new levels. There's a reason why the BOSU Balance Trainer is a staple in so many physical therapist offices and weight rooms: It just plain works.

In Part I, we start you off on your journey into *Weights on the BOSU Balance Trainer* by explaining what the BOSU Balance Trainer is, why and how you should use it, and why weights are necessary. We also answer some FAQs. We then prepare you to get into the workouts by providing some common-sense information, a recommendation to see your doctor and basic goal setting before you begin. Jason also talks in-depth about his rehabilitation on the BOSU Balance Trainer after a serious sports injury.

Part II starts off with some BOSU Balance Trainer basics, and then lets you practice with the BOSU Balance Trainer before explaining why and how you should diligently practice your form to build up a foundation to make your exercises safer and more effective. Once you're ready, we dive into the Basic and Advanced Programs, which are designed to build muscle, shred your core, develop outstanding agility and balance, train your entire

body for sports conditioning and build explosive power and strength. We also include a section on maintaining your physique after completing the Basic and Advanced programs.

Over 40 challenging and exciting exercises are described and illustrated in Part III. They're complemented by some "extra credit" advanced moves to supplement the program, as well as a few of our favorite extreme exercises to perform on the BOSU Balance Trainer. These are some of our favorite total-body moves to activate nearly every muscle from your fingertips to your toes.

The Appendix contains illustrated, step-by-step instructions for warm-ups and stretches to help you heal more quickly, develop flexibility and work your muscles through a full range of motion. Finally, you'll learn a little bit more about Jason and Brett.

So get ready, sit back and enjoy the ride. Using a BOSU Balance Trainer is going to be a different experience, one you're sure to find demanding and exhilarating. Even better? You'll absolutely love the results.

# What Is a BOSU Balance Trainer?

The BOSU Balance Trainer is a fitness and rehab device that debuted in 2000 with a rigid base attached to an inflated rubber hemisphere, or dome. It looks like a stability ball cut down the middle. "BOSU" is an acronym that originally stood for "BOth Sides Up," referencing the way the BOSU Balance Trainer can be positioned dome-side down or dome-side up. Recently, the phrase behind the acronym BOSU has been updated slightly to align more with the active participation that a practitioner has with the apparatus: "BOth Sides Utilized." The BOSU Balance Trainer isn't just passively "Up"—in order to provide the foundation for strengthening and toning bodies, it has to be actively "Utilized."

# BOSU Balance Trainer Models

As of this writing, there are four different models available, each varying slightly in size and construction: BOSU Balance Trainer, BOSU Pro Balance Trainer, BOSU Home Balance Trainer, BOSU Sport Balance Trainer.

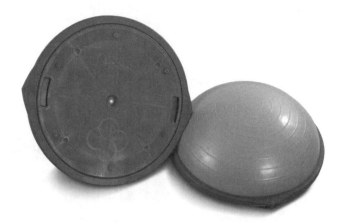

The most robust of the bunch is the BOSU Pro Balance Trainer, which features the largest arc of the dome at 65cm (inflation may vary) and is designed for enhanced durability with commercial-grade materials. The most expensive of the bunch, the Pro version was also made available in pink, with a portion of the proceeds going to breast cancer research.

The BOSU Balance Trainer is the standard model and features the same diameter as the Pro version (55cm) but a lower height (25cm) when inflated. Crafted from durable materials, this is often the most common apparatus found in athletic facilities all over the world.

The BOSU Home Balance Trainer is geared for home use and crafted for that purpose. It's the most inexpensively priced of the full 55cm models. The height remains unchanged from the standard model, 25cm.

The most compact and lightest version is the affordably priced BOSU Sport Balance Trainer.

Eschewing the molded black base, this sleeker, streamlined version still sports a flat, stable base opposite an inflated dome, yet is smaller and easily portable.

We've found the BOSU Balance Trainer to be an extraordinary device when recovering from injuries, working on nagging issues, getting a great workout quickly and increasing general body awareness. Combined with weights, all of these activities are compounded and intensified, creating an awesome workout.

# Why BOSU Balance Trainer?

In many ways the term "balance trainer" is apt, though it doesn't do it justice in the long run. The easiest way to describe the experience is to relate it to a very common activity. Take running. When you run on the road, you know the feel, you understand the cadence and you expect certain things. Try running on a trampoline, sand or water and all of a sudden nothing makes sense anymore. Your muscles don't fire the same way, your feet don't plant the same way and you actually have to think about and concentrate on the simplest activity. When stability is compromised, every movement requires myriad supporting muscles to be drawn into play in order to keep your body as centered as possible and prevent falling.

# Two Sides

The duality of the BOSU Balance Trainer's instability has led to its popularity. Its unstable surfaces have allowed trainers and practitioners to use it for a variety of purposes, including rehabilitation, no/low-impact cardio, strength training, balance training and even weight training.

With the BOSU Balance Trainer's dome-side up (a.k.a. Soft-Side Up, The Squish), the squishy blue half-orb can be used from a multitude of angles for stepping, standing, squatting, sitting, crunching and a whole lot of other activities. We'll explain these in "Getting on the BOSU Balance Trainer" on page 32 and then kick it up a notch by adding weights throughout the programs. When performing exercises on the dome's uniquely unstable surface, the black base lies flat on the floor to stabilize the entire device.

With the dome-side down, the base (a.k.a. Hard-Side Up, The Tray) creates a platform with a flat surface that can accommodate placement of hands, feet, knees or posterior—and nearly any combination thereof—to perform exercises, stretches, twists and lifts to strengthen and tone. The base allows for an interesting juxtaposition: a flat and relatively stable surface for performing unstable training. Hands or feet placed on the flat base in the upward position aren't subject to the pronation or supination that they'd undergo when placed on the half-dome surface.

The BOSU Balance Trainer excels in providing instability for enhanced total-body training. Take a push-up, one of the most standard bodyweight movements. Doing a push-up on a BOSU Balance Trainer, whether dome-side down or dome-side up, is more than a new experience—each is a unique exercise that completely changes the symphony of muscles required to complete this most basic of movements. Hands, wrists, shoulders, chest, back, core, arms—all these muscle groups are activated for not only the vertical up-and-down motion of the standard push-up, but recruited to work on all other axes or planes of movement caused by the instability of the dome deforming, rolling and pitching.

Like most great ideas and inventions that become a part of our daily lives, there's nothing inherently magical about the BOSU Balance Trainer—the genius is purely in its simplicity and adaptability. The BOSU Balance Trainer allows you to take existing exercises, lifts, twists and functional athletic movements, apply them to the apparatus and create entirely different workouts that stress and tax your muscles in new ways. Quite simply, it's a fantastic addition to any athlete's workout regimen.

# First Usage

Whoa.

Yes, that's the phrase nearly everyone utters when they step on either side of the BOSU Balance Trainer for the first time. Why? Because our brain always demands one thing above all others of our muscles: balance. Every position we put our bodies in during locomotion requires that equilibrium is somewhat maintained so that the brain can understand the spatial relationships and fire muscles accordingly to keep the body in motion. At rest, it's even easier to test: Just lean back in your chair a little bit; when you reach the point of unbalance, your brain will fire off the necessary muscles to attempt to keep you from falling.

Tied closely to that primal "fight or flight" instinct is the brain's need to be centered in order to handle whatever comes next. Training in an unstable environment on multiple changing planes helps to build strength, flexibility and a mind-body awareness that allows a wider range of movement and muscular activation. It even enhances athletic ability to perform complex maneuvers. Picture a skier landing a complex freestyle trick or a football receiver making an amazing catch at full speed, in the air and seemingly contorted. If you train purely in a linear fashion, these moves are beyond your reach.

Strength training on a BOSU Balance Trainer is far from a controlled, linear series of exercises—it maximizes multi-plane movements while muscles are under tension to deliver incredible strengthening and toning results you just can't achieve while lying flat on a bench. Period.

Now, if you've never done any type of unbalanced training before, you'll need to take it slow and develop multi-lateral stability in your muscles and joints. We assure you that *Weights on the BOSU Balance Trainer* is no joke and can be quite difficult at first.

## Mind-Body Connection

A fancy phrase used to describe awareness of your own body, muscles, movements and reactions is "kinesthetic awareness." As we age, this musculoskeletal and mental connection often declines, though hope is not lost! Kinesthetic awareness is trainable, and the BOSU Balance Trainer can help you reconnect with your body.

This leads to our next fancy word: "proprioception." Proprioception describes how your body reacts and responds to external forces to keep your joints in the correct position. When standing on the BOSU Balance Trainer, all your muscles are forced to contract to keep your joints in the proper position.

Don't think this is a big deal? Quick test: Stand on one foot with your other foot off the ground and close your eyes. Now just try to stand there for as long as you can. You see, in normal circumstances, we need vision to help us balance—this is natural. Closing your eyes makes you need to be aware of your muscles, and you need to actually focus on the balancing, with only your muscles reacting to the way your body is positioned. For most people this is incredibly difficult. The BOSU Balance Trainer takes this concept to an entirely new level. Standing on the apparatus you'll soon become aware of just what's needed to maintain various body positions. After some practice you'll be able to control even the small muscles in your body. This added awareness and control will help in all manners of your daily life.

# Why Weights?

Simply put, for enhanced strength training and adding muscle size and definition, there's no more effective workout in the world than a weighted one. Weights encourage muscle building, fat loss, and stimulation and activation of various hormonal changes needed to turn your body into whatever you want. When paired with extremely effective bodyweight movements and then performed in multiple planes on a BOSU Balance Trainer, there's simply nothing as effective at developing athletic ability, functional strength and reshaping your physique.

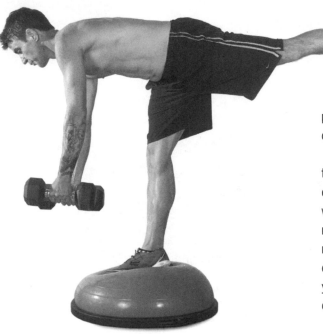

testosterone levels through supplementation. Adding weighted exercises to your workouts only increases your ability to strengthen and tone, especially when performed as part of a full-body routine like the one in this book.

Even the goal of fat loss is aided by weight training. Often people hoping to lose fat will engage in some form of cardio activity like jogging when, in truth, adding a weighted workout to their routine is a much better choice for delivering the results they seek even more quickly. We've developed the programs in this book to help you torch your fat with full-body workouts that are fast and challenging yet—dare we say—fun.

Contrast the toning or weight-loss goals with men or women who want to pack on as much muscle as possible. Again, weights are needed here, just with a much different emphasis on sets, reps, nutrition, rest and recovery. The workouts in this book are not designed for maximal muscle gain. Rather, they're focused on improved athletic performance, agility, balance, strength, toning, power and even endurance.

The main point to take away is that performing weighted workouts enhances our ability to get stronger, fitter and develop a leaner physique than relying on just cardiovascular activities. Combining weights with traditional bodyweight movements is a plus; adding in the extreme effectiveness of performing it on a BOSU Balance Trainer only amplifies the positive benefits. The real key is knowing what you want to achieve. This will help you define the parameters of which weights to use.

Want to create a lean, ripped body? Adding weights are the key.

Want to gain some muscle? Pick up some weights.

Want to simply lose fat? Combining weights with nearly any other form of training will amplify the fat-burning cycle by developing lean muscle.

Weighted workouts are the key to taking your strength and physique to the next level. The question you should really be asking yourself is, what do you actually want to do? Knowing your goal will help you decide the key points in your weight-training program.

For instance, women quite often want to "tone up" or create a long and lean look. Weights, even heavy ones, are great for this. Yes, women can and should lift weights; they're not going to excessively "bulk up" without drastically changing their

# Frequently Asked Questions

**Q.** What should I wear when I'm working out?

**A.** Any type of non-restrictive clothing is perfect. Many people like to use the BOSU Balance Trainer barefoot or with sneakers. We don't recommend socks as the dome surface can be slippery.

**Q.** What kind of weights should I use?

**A.** For nearly all the moves in this book, a weighted vest and a pair of dumbbells will suffice. With some slight modification of hand position, a medicine ball will do nicely as well. Here's a little list for cross-reference:

**DUMBBELLS:** Hand-held, balanced weights on opposite sides of a grip, 2.5 to over 85 pounds

**MEDICINE BALLS** (a.k.a. Med Ball, Exercise Ball, Fitness Ball): Usually the size and shape of a basketball, 5 to 25 pounds (heavier ones available by special order)

**BODY BARS:** 4-foot-long foam-covered weighted bars, 5 to 25 pounds

**WEIGHTED VEST:** A vest with built-in or adjustable weights to increase your bodyweight while keeping your hands free to perform exercises, 5 to 65 pounds

**ANKLE/WRIST WEIGHTS:** Flexible weighted bands designed to wrap around extremities and stay in place during movements; available in .5 to over 10 pounds.

**KETTLEBELLS:** Weighted bells with a handle, available in 2.5 to well over 100 pounds

**SHORT OLYMPIC BAR:** 5 feet long, 30 pounds

**STANDARD OLYMPIC BAR:** 7 feet long, 45 pounds

As you can see, there are plenty of options for your strength, ability and willingness to adapt some of the movements to utilize different hand positions to accommodate different-size and -shape weights.

*Please note:* This book only describes and illustrates the usage of dumbbells, medicine balls, weighted vests, ankle/wrist weights and body bars on specific movements. Use other weights and equipment at your own risk.

**Q.** How heavy should the weights I use be?

**A.** First off, you'll be starting without weights until you're comfortable with performing unbalanced exercises (see "Getting on the BOSU Balance Trainer" on page 32). When you're ready for weights, you'll start with very light weights and increase as you progress through the program. Weight should never be a static number. As you get stronger you should increase the amount you lift incrementally based on your comfort level and increases in strength. This progressive resistance is the key to making progress in all exercise programs. The moment you stop upping your weights is the moment you stop making gains. Sure, you can play with tempo or reps and sets and you'll see some progress with this, but nothing as quick as you would by increasing your weights.

Mind you, we'll be challenging you to increase your work capacity by going longer and harder as the workouts progress, but we want to emphasize that you should be using as heavy a weight as you can safely handle and perform each rep with proper form.

**Q.** I have an injury. Can I still work out?

**A.** See your doctor. Boring answer, but the truth. The workouts are rigorous and the addition of instability could make some very common injuries worse if you're not careful. The BOSU Balance Trainer is a great tool to use for rehab on many frequently injured body parts such as knees, ankles, back and hips, but it should be done under a doctor's supervision. We have no illusions that prescribing exercise is the answer to all injuries and would not think to give medical advice in those circumstances (or any; we're CPTs, not MDs). Above all else, be safe and see your doctor first before performing any demanding physical activity.

**Q.** I already work out at the gym. Would I get anything out of this?

**A.** Absolutely! The exercises and workouts here would make anyone a fitter person, not to mention a better athlete. Who can't use a stronger core, more balanced and stable musculature, and better body awareness?

**Q.** I hate working out. Why is this different?

**A.** Truth be told, it might not be. But it'll likely be more effective. We've found that most people who hate working out hate it for a very small set of reasons. Perhaps they aren't making progress or perhaps they don't like taking too long on an individual session. It might be that they feel insecure and don't know what to do. For a vast majority, the gym can be viewed as an inhospitable, menacing place where they feel overwhelmed by the atmosphere and the sheer magnitude of machines. They may even feel like they're being unfairly judged by other members. One of the goals with all our *7 Weeks to Fitness* books is to make working out and getting fit as simple and least overwhelming as possible. Getting fit is much more achievable when you can follow along with a plan and see your progress take shape.

We provide a step-by-step workout that gets fantastic results in minimal time. The principles here are the exact same principles we use in all of our successful programs. If you want to achieve something spectacular and you want to do it quickly, this is the place to be.

**Q.** I'm a runner. Will this help me?

**A.** Not only will this program help you, it's our humble assertion that it'll take your running to a whole new level. Brett and Jason are both "runners," albeit on different levels. Brett is an accomplished triathlete and marathoner who enjoys longer-distance running and incorporates as many quality weekly miles as possible into his regimen to keep his endurance up and his body lean. His running efficiency reached new heights when he started taking weight training seriously; strengthening the muscle groups that were less-used in his running regimen led to exponential gains in overall strength and vitality as well as minimizing injuries. Jason is a bit more of a "weekend warrior" type of runner; he's fast over short distances and is extremely effective at sports like football, rugby or basketball, yet not much of a long-distance runner. His exact quote during his first ultramarathon may have been "Just shoot me." Jason brings a whole other level of BOSU Balance Trainer experience to the table as he has suffered numerous injuries over the years at multiple different athletic endeavors,

from pushing cars to trail hill sprints. Using the programs and exercises outlined in this book, he has been able to rehab and do things he never thought he would do again...namely, run. Learn more about Jason's rehab experiences on page 27.

**Q.** How much time do I need, really?

**A.** It'll vary from person to person depending on how fit they are, but generally speaking you should be done with your warm-up, workout and cool-down in under 30 minutes. Look, we know everyone is busy and has hectic lives. We know we do! People need maximum results in minimal time. The programs are geared around just that. By working your total body through a series of supersets you can achieve maximal strengthening, toning and conditioning in less time.

**Q.** I want to tone up. Won't weights make me bulky?

**A.** No. Absolutely not. This is a common fear for women. Ask any man working out in the gym just how hard it is to get the "bulky" look. Most men crave bigger muscles, yet so few achieve it. Why? Diet. Muscle size is more a function of what and how you eat and not how you work out. Weights are the key to a healthy lifestyle, but how big you get depends on how much of the various macronutrients you eat. No, lifting weights without following a specific muscle-building nutrition plan won't make you bulky at all.

**Q.** What's the difference between a BOSU Balance Trainer and any other unstable surface I can exercise on?

**A.** We've been using a BOSU Balance Trainer for nearly a decade for conditioning, agility training, injury rehabilitation and developing sport-specific skills, so when it came to writing this book there was no question what apparatus we would recommend—the same one we've used ourselves. Let's make it clear that neither Jason nor Brett work for or are in any way compensated to choose BOSU-branded products for use in our training or with clients. We choose to use BOSU Balance Trainers because they're extremely effective, safe and dependable. There are plenty of other types of choices that can be made regarding exercise equipment—it's important to pick the right tool for the job with confidence that it'll deliver. In our opinion, when it comes to unstable workouts like those listed in this book, the clear-cut answer is to use and recommend a BOSU Balance Trainer.

**Q.** I just had a baby. Can I do this workout?

**A.** See your doctor first. This answer also applies to "I just had surgery," "I just pulled a muscle," "I just completed my first Spartan Race and I still can't look at a cargo net without weeping a little...." No matter what your starting point is, getting a check-up from your doc should always be the first step.

**Q.** I have weak knees (or ankles, lower back, hips, etc.) and want to use unstable workouts to strengthen them. Can I jump right in?

**A.** While unstable workouts are one of the best ways to rehab many weaknesses or injuries resulting from weak joints or body parts that are responsible for taking a lot of impact, you should never "jump in" to any advanced program after an injury or chronic soreness or instability. Here's the progression everyone should follow when building up to an advanced routine:

• Stable exercises on a flat surface, bodyweight only

• Stable exercises using light weights that allow you to keep proper form throughout the entire range of motion; add additional weights as you progress in strength and comfort with the movements

• Unstable exercises on a safe, durable, quality apparatus like the BOSU Balance Trainer, using only bodyweight and assistance from a spotter as needed

• Unstable exercises with light weights that allow you to maintain perfect form; progress to heavier weights only when you can complete all the desired reps with proper form

Just remember: Using heavier weights with bad form is a complete waste of time and results in poor gains, injuries and more often than not looking like a fool. Struggling to push up too much weight can make anyone look like a turtle trying to get it on with a fire hydrant—not a pleasant sight.

# Before You Begin

If we haven't beaten you over the head with the "see your doctor first before starting any workout program" phrasing, let's just give you five practical examples of why seeing a doctor first is the most important step toward getting in shape:

1. You may be in better shape than you realize—it happens every day. How many times do you hear a co-worker say, "I got a clean bill of health, my doc says I have the heart of a teenager!"

2. You may find out you have to switch your goals and fix a potential problem. Let's face it, humans were given brains in order to solve things—we love to fix stuff. Your doctor may give you some professional insight into some fixes that your body may need, whether proactively, to prevent something, or reactively, to take care of now. Do you know your cholesterol levels? Do you even know what they should be? How about your blood pressure, lung and heart function? All these are very easy things for a trained medical profession to test for—this is why they're professionals!

3. Use your doctor's visit as a chance to play show and tell. No, wait, that's a bad idea. How about using your visit as a chance for some Q&A. Engage your doc and ask some of the questions from #2 above. Ask what your weight should be, things you should be aware of based on your medical history and that of your family. She's the one with the clipboard in her hand. Many times there's answers in there that you need to ask for. Be vocal—you're the one paying for the visit! Your health and well-being are your responsibility, and sometimes you won't get that extra bit of important information unless you ask.

4. There could be something serious that you can't ignore. It's the elephant in the room but it needs to be said: You need to know if there's anything wrong BEFORE you push yourself. Humans are messy and complicated, just like the wiring of a 1962 Jaguar E-Type. Both require being brought to a professional to decipher, diagnose and repair.

5. It may prevent you from spinning your wheels while trying to reach your goals. Can't gain muscle or lose weight no matter how hard you try? The problem may be no bigger than the tip of your pinkie finger—your pituitary gland's function may be out of whack. Maybe your thyroid is operating at hyper- or hypothyroid levels? Are you anemic? What about any other vitamin deficiencies? The answer is most likely hidden inside of you and you just don't know until you get checked out. Go to a professional and decipher your own internal *DaVinci Code*.

One last time for the lawyers: Prior to beginning this or any physical fitness regimen, it's recommended that you visit a licensed physician and receive a clean bill of health before you proceed.

# Rehab on the BOSU: Jason's Experience

So far we've spent quite a bit of time explaining how the BOSU Balance Trainer is a great workout tool. We'll spend even more time showing how you can achieve the results you've always wanted by combining it with weights. If you've been following along and start doing the workouts, we're sure you'll be convinced too.

But truth be told, that's not what initially sold us, particularly Jason, on the BOSU Balance Trainer.

**JASON:** In 2006 I tore my Achilles tendon training for basketball. It wasn't a full tear, but something referred to as a partial rupture. The pain was real, the not-being-able-to-walk was real and the scary "will I ever get back to walking, let alone sports?" question was absolutely real. I had never experienced anything like this and didn't know what to do.

I was put in a walking boot for three months, which did very little to actually help the problem. I was beyond disheartened. After the walking boot, the docs started the rehab. It was in rehab that I first saw the BOSU Balance Trainer. It was tucked away in the corner near the section with balls and bands. The physiotherapist sat me down and walked me through the plan. We were getting going a bit and she pointed over to the BOSU Balance Trainer and said, "And then we'll get to that, but you aren't ready for it yet."

What? Not ready? Are you kidding me? I was ready for anything that would get me back on the basketball court. I protested, explained that I was, indeed, ready. She held her ground. She plainly said that:

1. If I wasn't smart, I could re-injure the Achilles;
2. There was no way that I was ready to step on the BOSU Balance Trainer on the first day. My body (not my Achilles, mind you) was not aware enough to handle it.

Are you kidding me? There was no way I was going to stand for that! So we went through the session, we did the intro rehab, scheduled bi-weekly follow-ups for the next two months and then I was on my way. What was the first thing I did after leaving the physiotherapist's office? Head to a sports store and buy a BOSU Balance Trainer.

Seriously, how hard could it be? Of course I was ready! I was a physically fit 26-year-old male who played basketball four to six times a week. I was active, I knew my body and I lifted weights. If anyone was ready, it was me. Even so, I thought I was going to be clever, do it smart. I was going to start with my non-injured foot and do the rehab exercises just to be sure. Less than 30 seconds in and I was already on the floor! Two minutes in and, while I didn't admit it, I knew I wasn't ready.

How in the hell? The physiotherapist absolutely nailed it. So what did happen? Well, truth be told, all my weights, all my basketball and sports training didn't actually develop my balance. It turns out that balance is a physical skill just like any other. It has to be trained to be developed, you just don't "get it for free" doing other things. I really did need to take it slow, particularly with my injured Achilles.

Fast forward six weeks. It was my first day with my injured Achilles on the BOSU Balance Trainer in front of my physiotherapist. I was nervous, but she barely flinched. After all, it wasn't her Achilles! The hard honest truth is that it was more difficult and painful than I can describe. Sessions 2–4 were uncomfortable, but increasingly less so. My balance and flexibility continually got better. In the course of a quick three weeks, my Achilles went from an estimated 30% strength and function to 60%, more quickly than the previous five months combined! For the first time since tearing it, I actually thought I might play basketball again.

However, I couldn't get ahead of myself. Like most things, the initial gains and recovery slowed and eventually plateaued. When I finished physiotherapy, my estimated strength and function in the Achilles was approximately 80%.

But 30% to 80% in about three months? SOLD! I continued to use the BOSU Balance Trainer nearly every day until I got to about 90% and stepped on the court for the first time since tearing it. I was 100% convinced of its effectiveness and continued to use it in my daily rehab regime. It became even more important when I started playing basketball again. I'm in love with my BOSU Balance Trainer.

Six years later I don't use my BOSU Balance Trainer on a daily basis for rehab anymore, though I do use it about once a week. I also don't play nearly as much basketball as I once did. If I were still playing four to six times a week, I know I'd be using the BOSU Balance Trainer nearly as often as I did when I first rehabbed.

One last point: While I was rehabbing my right leg (the side with the torn Achilles), I decided it'd be smart to also train my left leg with similar exercises. I didn't struggle nearly as much with this, but it did take time for me to acclimate to the balance stresses I wasn't

used to. But I persisted and, when I finally did step on the basketball court, I was quicker, more aware of my feet and overall body placement—I was a better basketball player. It didn't show in the first few weeks because I needed to work my torn Achilles back into game shape, but when I did, it was clear I was not only back, but also a better version of my basketball-playing self.

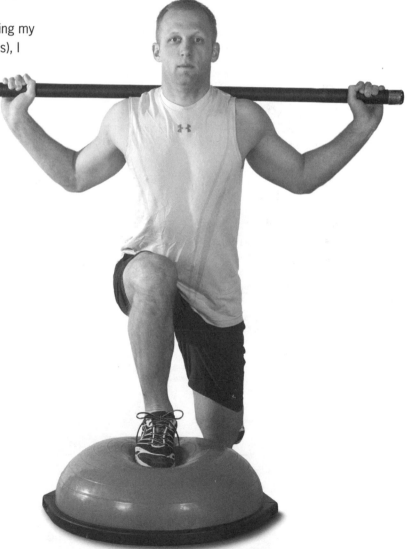

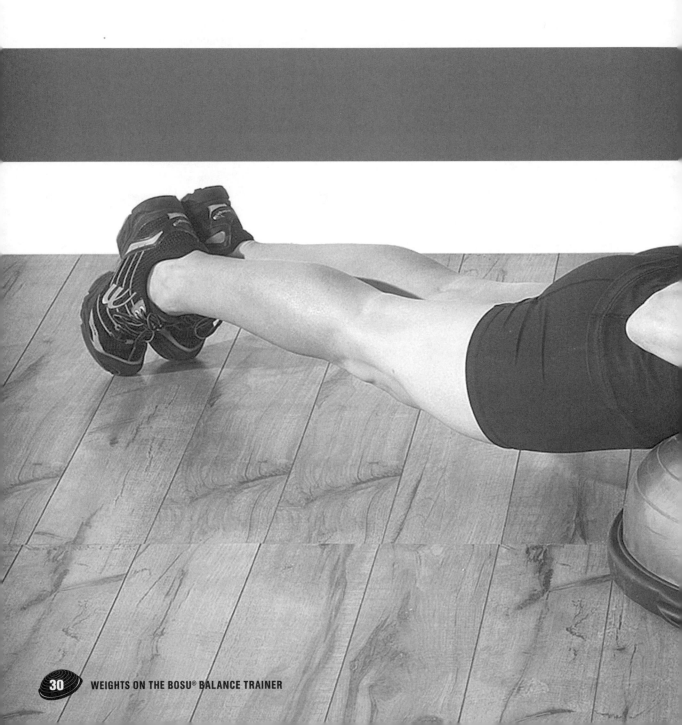

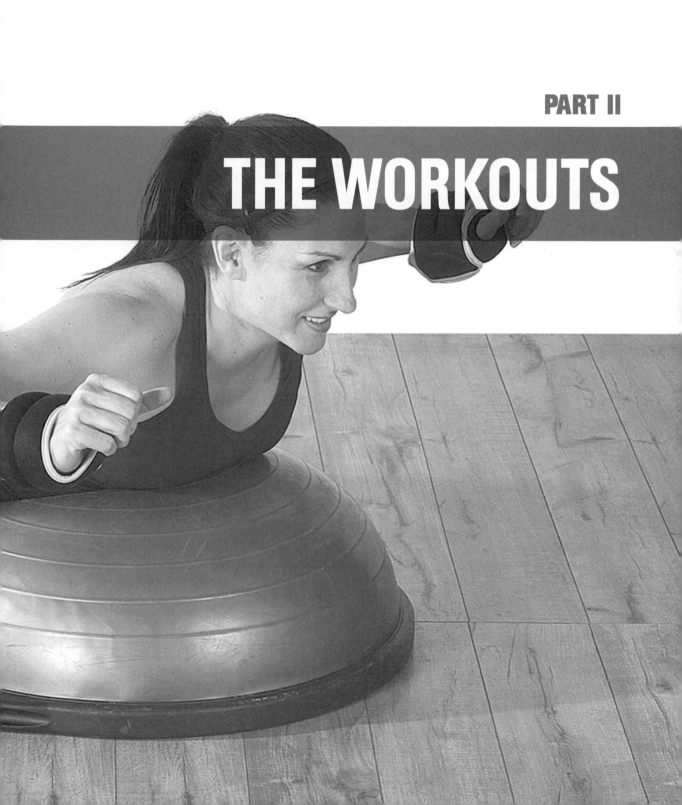

# Getting on the BOSU Balance Trainer

If you've gotten this far, it's a fair assumption that you know what a BOSU Balance Trainer is and you've either purchased your own or belong to a gym that has a few. We'll go so far as to say you've most likely already spent at least a little bit of time on one, whether standing, squatting, sitting or crunching on it. If so, you can skip ahead. For those who are new to the BOSU Balance Trainer and have yet to give it a go, here are some tips to using your new piece of equipment properly and safely. Yes, accidents do happen and the nature of an unbalanced workout can raise the possibility if you're not fully aware of what you're doing and how you're performing each exercise. Use these pointers to help keep your workouts safe and fun.

- Make sure your BOSU Balance Trainer is clean and dry. Both the rubber dome and flat base can be slippery when wet, dirty or even oily from repeated use with bare hands, feet, forearms, etc.
- Wear soft-soled shoes that have clean treads (see above) or go barefoot. Wearing socks on the domed side can be slippery.
- Step carefully—don't jump on the BOSU Balance Trainer until you're extremely familiar with the unstable surface. Along those lines, remember that the balance trainer is not a trampoline.
- Learn to stand before you can walk, or at least learn to stand and balance before you try exercises. Practice stepping forward onto the BOSU Balance Trainer dome-side up with one foot and then stepping back off a few times to get a feel for how the dome deforms under your foot. When you're ready, step forward with one foot followed by the other, holding onto a spotter or a secure railing until you have your balance. Adjust your feet so that the positioning is secure, and practice

standing with perfect posture: head up, back straight and shoulders back.
- Once you've mastered dome-side up, flip the BOSU Balance Trainer over and get comfortable stepping on and maintaining your balance with the flat-side up. They're both entirely different experiences to get used to, so take your time and make sure you're steady before adding any movements, exercises and weights.

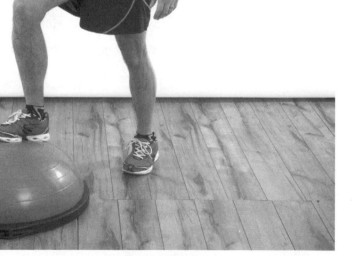

# Creating the Proper BOSU Balance Trainer Foundation

As we mentioned in "Getting on the BOSU Balance Trainer" (page 32), it's important to learn the basics before you progress to more advanced moves. In this case, it's extremely necessary to become proficient in performing basic exercises on the BOSU Balance Trainer with flawless form before moving on to more complicated, compound movements (multi-muscle and multi-joint, usually referred to as full-body) and then adding weights. Why? Well, for three main reasons:

**1. Bad form results in bad results:** You won't be targeting the proper muscles that the exercise or program is designated for if your form is off. For example, the angle of your torso when lifting a weight makes all the difference between an incline chest press, which develops your pectoral muscles, and a front shoulder press, which works your deltoids.

**2. Bad form results in injury:** No surprise here. When you put your body in an awkward position (more on that in #3), you're more prone to pulling, tearing or breaking things that have no business being incorporated into that movement. For example, performing squats with your knees bowed inward more often than not results in knee strain, pain and even damaging your meniscus.

**3. Bad form results in you looking like an idiot:** Let's just be honest, anyone who falls off a ball is going to illicit a snicker from even their closest friends and workout partners—not to mention the rest of the gym faithful! (Of course, that's as long as you don't get hurt; no one should ever laugh about that.) All kidding aside, it's acceptable to struggle with a new and difficult exercise until you get it right, especially when it's a challenging unbalanced movement. It's another thing altogether when you watch someone struggling through an exercise with too heavy a weight or with really bad form. Unfortunately, unless someone corrects them or they do a little online or written research or "gym reconnaissance," they'll stick to the same improper form and wind up a candidate for #1 or #2 above.

**TIP:** Gym reconnaissance is used by many, but sometimes it's a recipe for disaster. Just because that gal over there with the amazing abs does her medicine ball wood chop in her own way, it doesn't mean her form is perfect. Do some research online or pick up a book and make sure you know what you're doing before you adopt her style. On the flip side, if you see someone absolutely struggling and making the exercise look more like a battle than a movement, you should probably not adopt their style. Even difficult exercises should be controlled, normally fluid motions.

In this section, we start off with the basic building blocks for all of the more-advanced programs. It's extremely important that you develop a solid, strong foundation by learning proper exercise form before attempting ANY of these exercises on the BOSU Balance Trainer.

Our goals for creating a proper BOSU Balance Trainer foundation:

**Goal 1:** Begin with and master stable exercises on a flat surface using your bodyweight only.

**Goal 2:** On a stable surface, add light weights that allow you to keep proper form throughout the entire range of motion. Add additional weights as you progress in strength and comfort with the movements.

**Goal 3:** Carefully practice exercises on the BOSU Balance Trainer using only bodyweight and assistance from a spotter as needed.

**Goal 4:** Perform unstable exercises with light weights that allow you to maintain perfect form. Progress to heavier weights only when you can complete all the desired reps with proper form.

Depending on athletic ability, previous workout experience, strength and coordination, some individuals can progress through all of these four goals in four sets of one workout, each set of exercises moving up one goal. Many individuals will need to perform a week's worth of workouts or more to feel completely comfortable using weights on the BOSU Balance Trainer and that's no problem at all! Simply perform as many workouts or weeks as you need to progress to the point where you can perform the weighted workouts on the BOSU Balance Trainer as described in Goal 4. There's no rush to complete each of the goals. The workouts in this book, from Basic to Advanced, are designed to be used as often as you want and for as long as you want to develop and maintain your fitness and physique.

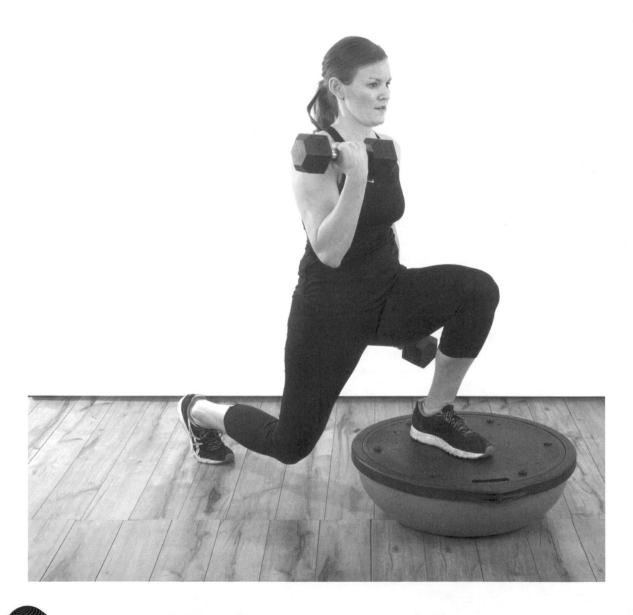

# Preparing for the Workouts

In order to achieve the results you're working on by using the programs in this book, it's very important to be ready for the challenge and know your limits. We know we've said this before, but when you begin any new exercise program, it's imperative that you talk with your doctor first and make sure you're healthy enough to participate in physical strength training and conditioning.

Once you begin the Basic or Advanced Strength Training on the BOSU Balance Trainer program, perform it at your own pace and within your personal level of fitness. If you're new to working out, especially balance-based training, or returning to exercise after some time off, be sure to take your time and take it easy for the first two weeks to allow your muscles to adjust to the new workload and reduce post-workout soreness. DOMS is the acronym for "delayed onset muscle soreness" and the simple reality is that the soreness you experience 24, 48 or more hours after pushing a workout too hard will hamper, limit or completely sabotage your program. You have plenty of time to get in the groove with this program, so take your time and work your way into it!

This may come as a shock, but no one's perfect at every exercise when they get started—usually far from it! Even after some practice, you still won't be a pro at every movement. Some exercises may come naturally while others feel completely foreign, and almost all unbalanced exercises take a long time to master. Multi-joint, multi-muscle movements like squats are already complicated and difficult to master on the flat ground; when you perform them on a BOSU Balance Trainer, they're a much more demanding yet rewarding exercise. It's extremely important to keep working on perfecting the form and get stronger along the way. Don't give up and sit out an exercise if you can't do it—make the investment in yourself and learn the proper form for each move. You'll only reap the benefits.

If you feel extremely fatigued or have an uncomfortable level of pain and soreness, take two to three days off from the workout. Some muscle fatigue and soreness is to be expected and you can continue to exercise carefully when you're a little tired or sore. Any sharp pain, pinches or throbbing aches in joints is not to be ignored; if the discomfort or pain persists, seek the advice of a medical professional. If you feel any sensation in a joint or muscle that makes you say "uh-oh," then stop immediately, rest and assess whether it's a serious injury that needs medical attention.

Due to the nature of a full-body, unstable workout routine, you'll be lifting, pushing and pressing your entire bodyweight. It's very important that you focus on proper form and utilize the proper muscles to complete each exercise. This means no cheating by arching your back on push-ups or allowing your knees to bow in during squats— you're only cheating yourself. Every proper-form rep just gets you closer to your goals!

If you have a pre-existing condition like joint instability or a muscular imbalance, make sure you recognize any physical limitations, take your time and work your way up slowly while focusing on training with good form. It's far more important to be careful with nagging injuries than it is to worry about completing all the exercises in any specified amount of time. Performing the exercises with proper form will help you to build strength, flexibility and balance as well as improve your sports performance—but not if you ignore the warning signs and hurt yourself. If pain or soreness persists, please see a medical professional.

The exercises in this book were designed specifically to be performed on the BOSU Balance Trainer, and we only recommend using a licensed product. If you choose to use other unstable surfaces, be smart and safe—don't take any chances with unsafe equipment, and make sure you're properly trained to use any equipment before you start a workout. Always be aware of your surroundings and make sure you have plenty of room to execute moves safely without hitting or tripping over other objects.

# Warming Up & Stretching

Properly warming up the body prior to any activity is very important, as is stretching post-workout. Please note that warming up and stretching are two completely different things: A warm-up routine should be done before stretching so that your muscles are more pliable and able to be stretched efficiently. You should not "warm up" by stretching; you simply don't want to push, pull or stretch cold muscles.

Prior to warming up, your muscles are significantly less flexible. Think of pulling a rubber band out of a freezer: If you stretch it forcefully before it has a chance to warm up, you'll likely tear it. Stretching cold muscles can cause a significantly higher rate of muscle strains and even injuries to joints that rely on those muscles for alignment.

It's crucial to raise your body temperature prior to beginning a workout. In order to prevent injury, such as a muscle strain, you want to loosen up your muscles and joints before you begin the actual exercise movement. A good warm-up before your workout should slowly raise your core body temperature, heart rate and breathing. Before jumping into the workout, you must increase blood flow to all working areas of the body. This augmented blood flow will transport more oxygen and nutrients to the muscles being worked. The warm-up will also increase the range of motion of your joints.

Another goal is to focus your mental awareness and body proprioception. You've heard that meditation requires being present in the "now." The same is true for a demanding exercise routine. Being totally present and focused will help you perform better and avoid injury.

A proper warm-up should consist of light physical activity (such as walking, jogging, stationary biking or jumping jacks) and only take 5–10 minutes to complete. Your individual fitness level and the activity determine how hard and how long you should go but, generally speaking, the average person should build up to a light sweat during warm-ups. You want to prepare your body for activity, not fatigue it.

A warm-up should be done in these stages:

- **Gentle Mobility:** Easy movements that get your joints moving freely, like standing arm raises, arm and shoulder circles, neck rotations, and trunk twists.
- **Pulse Raising:** Gentle, progressive, aerobic activity that starts the process of raising your heart rate, like jumping jacks, skipping rope or running in place.
- **Specific Mobility:** This begins working the joints and muscles that will be used during the activity. Perform dynamic movements to prepare your body for your upcoming full-body workout. These movements are done more rapidly than the gentle mobility movements—envision a swimmer before a race or a weightlifter before a big lift. Dynamic movements should raise the heart rate, loosen specific joints and muscles, and get you motivated for your workout.

Stretching should generally be done after a workout. It'll help you reduce muscle soreness from the workout, increase range of motion and flexibility within a joint or muscle, and prepare your body for any future workouts. Stretching immediately post-exercise while your muscles are still warm allows your muscles to return to their full range of motion (which gives you more flexibility gains) and reduces the chance of injury or fatigue in the hours or days after an intense workout. It's important to remember that even when you're warm and loose, you should never "bounce" during stretching. Keep your movements slow and controlled.

To recap, you should warm up for 5–10 minutes, perform your workout, and then stretch for 5–10 minutes. We've included a few warm-up exercises and stretches that specifically target the muscles used in each workout (page 106).

# Avoiding Injuries

As we covered earlier in the FAQs (page 21), bodyweight strength training combined with unstable exercises and weights is an incredibly efficient way to build strength, flexibility and balance as well as develop a lean, ripped physique. Let's be honest, though; none of us is perfect. Due to years of improper posture, sports injuries or even weak musculature, we all have imbalances that can affect proper form and even put us on the fast track to injury. In addition, jumping into a new exercise routine too quickly or doing the exercises with improper form can exacerbate any pre-existing injury. Unstable surfaces make it even more precarious for first-timers or those coming back after a layoff. This is why we recommend starting on a flat surface without weights before stepping up to the BOSU Balance Trainer and adding in weights.

Throughout the routine, you should expect to experience mild soreness and fatigue, especially when you're just getting started. The feeling of your muscles being "pumped" and the fatigue of an exhausting workout should be expected. These are positive feelings.

On the other hand, any sharp pain, muscle spasm or numbness is a warning sign that you need to stop and not push yourself any harder. Some small muscle groups may fatigue more quickly because they're often overlooked in other workouts. Your hands and forearms are doing a tremendous amount of work and can easily tire out. If you feel you can't grip or support yourself with your hands anymore, take a rest. It's far better than slipping and getting hurt.

Here are a few other symptoms to watch for: sore elbows, shoulder (rotator cuff) pain and stiff neck. Sore elbows are usually a sign that you're locking out your elbows when your arms are fully extended; remember to keep a slight bend in your elbows. Pain in the rotator cuff can be caused by poor form or a hand position that's too wide while doing push-ups or overhead presses. A stiff neck can result from straining your neck throughout the movement; try to keep your neck loose and flexible. If any of these pains persists, it's imperative that you seek medical advice. Be smart, stay safe and take your time adjusting to the program!

# Basic Program

DO NOT LET THE NAME FOOL YOU. If you're new to BOSU Balance Trainer training, the Basic program is more appropriately named "For the love of god, don't skip me!" The only thing basic about this is that we want you to become comfortable with both the BOSU Balance Trainer and how you react to the balance stresses placed on your body. These are the "basic" elements needed to go further and successfully perform the more-advanced exercises in the Advanced program.

As said, the Basic program is about learning how to use, control and balance on both sides of the BOSU Balance Trainer. You'll become comfortable standing on either the dome or the disc side with one or both feet. You'll understand where to place your feet and hands when doing the exercises. You'll get a sense for how you respond to all the exercises, where you can improve and how you can apply more or less stress. The bottom line is you'll actually be in tune with your body.

Both the Basic and Advanced programs are structured the same but with much different exercises. We'll focus on the core movements here and get to the fancier stuff in the Advanced program.

The actual program is simple. There'll be a list of exercises with either a timeframe or given reps. Complete each exercise for the prescribed time or reps in order before moving on to the next exercise. Once you've completed all the exercises in order, that's one set. Continue until you've completed all the sets. Like we said—simple!

Remember the goals we outlined in "Creating the Proper BOSU Balance Trainer Foundation" on page 34? Well, here's where we put them to the test. Start by performing each exercise on a flat, stable surface before adding light weights, then progress to performing them on the BOSU Balance Trainer before adding the weights back in. Like all progressive programs, as you get stronger you can add more weight and/or reps, and/or extend the duration of timed exercises. When you're really ready to step it up a notch, reduce or eliminate the rest between sets and perform each round as an 11-move superset to build endurance and rev your metabolism to torch fat while developing the strength and flexibility the BOSU Balance Trainer is famous for delivering.

Take your time. If you can't perform all the reps without taking a break, take the break. If you can't go the full time stated at first, take a quick breather. This isn't an easy workout, and it only

| | MONDAY | TUESDAY | WEDNESDAY | THURSDAY | FRIDAY | SAT/SUN |
|---|---|---|---|---|---|---|
| Perform the designated workout routine on the corresponding day noted on the chart below. Rest for 1 to 2 minutes between each round. | | | | | | |
| WEEK 1 | Lower Body | Core | Upper Body | Core | Lower Body | OFF |
| WEEK 2 | Upper Body | Core | Lower Body | Core | Upper Body | OFF |
| WEEK 3 | Lower Body/Core | Upper Body | OFF | Lower Body | Upper Body/Core | OFF |
| WEEK 4 | Full Body 1 | Lower Body/Core | OFF | Upper Body/Core | Full Body 2 | OFF |
| WEEK 5 | Lower Body/Core | Full Body 1 | Core | Full Body 2 | Upper Body/Core | OFF |
| WEEK 6 | Full Body 1 | Lower Body | Core | Full Body 2 | Lower Body | OFF |
| WEEK 7 | Full Body 1 | Full Body 2 | Core | Full Body 1 | Full Body 2 | OFF |

gets more difficult as you progress. Stick with it and you'll get there!

Some parting words of advice from two guys who have been through it: Give it your all. You owe it to yourself to give everything you have. We know there'll be frustration initially, progress might be slow and you might feel like you'll never be able to do it. KEEP GOING! Each workout is going to get easier, each day you'll get better and each session on the BOSU Balance Trainer you'll find new strength you didn't think you had. Give the program time to work and yourself time to adjust. If you do, you'll accomplish more than you ever thought you could and you'll change in ways you didn't think possible. There's nothing magical about the BOSU Balance Trainer, though there is something magical about desire, persistence and dedication.

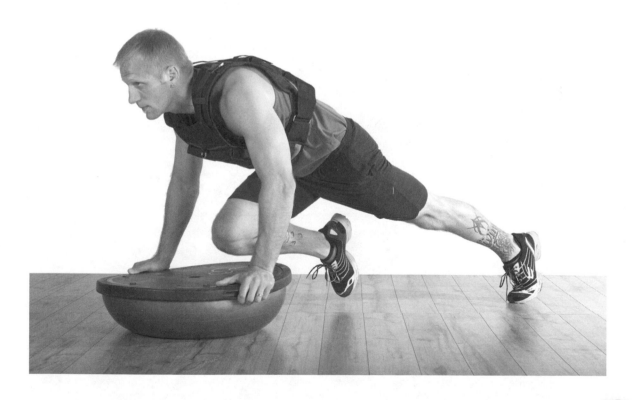

## BASIC PROGRAM: FULL BODY 1

| EXERCISE | REPS/TIME |
|---|---|
| Push-Up *(page 55)*/alternate sets with Toe-Balance Push-Up *(page 56)* | 5 |
| Plank *(page 79)* | 0:30 |
| Squat *(page 73)* | 8 |
| Mason Twist *(page 81)* | 8 |
| Mountain Climber *(page 86)* | 8 each leg |
| Back Extension *(page 83)*/alternate sets with Reverse Fly *(page 72)* | 6 |
| Burpee *(page 87)* | 5 |
| Ab Crunch *(page 82)* | 12 |
| Diamond Push-Up *(page 57)* | 5 |
| Lunge *(page 76)* | 5 each leg |
| Front Row *(page 70)* | 6 |
| Do 3 rounds total | |

## BASIC PROGRAM: FULL BODY 2

| EXERCISE | REPS/TIME |
|---|---|
| Diamond Push-Up, dome-side down *(p. 57)* | 5 |
| Goblet Squat *(page 73)* | 6 |
| Overhead Press *(page 65)*/alternate sets with Triceps Extension *(page 66)* | 6 |
| Bounce-Up *(page 61)* | 4 |
| Burpee *(page 87)* | 6 |
| Step-Up with Dumbbell Curl *(page 75)*/alternate sets with Triceps Kickback *(page 67)* | 6 each side |
| Plank Row *(page 80)* | 4 each side |
| Hip Raise/Glute Bridge *(page 85)* | 12 |
| Lunge with Dumbbell *(page 76)* | 6 |
| Bird Dog *(page 84)* | 8 |
| Front Raise *(page 69)*/alternate sets with Lateral Raise *(page 68)* | 6 |
| Do 3 rounds total | |

## BASIC PROGRAM: LOWER BODY

| EXERCISE | REPS/TIME |
|---|:---:|
| Squat *(page 73)* | 8 |
| Step-Up with Dumbbell Curl *(page 75)* | 8 |
| Squat with Overhead Press *(page 74)* | 4 |
| Back Extension *(page 83)* | 12 |
| Lunge *(page 76)* | 6 each side |
| Lunge with Dumbbell *(page 76)* | 6 each side |
| Bird Dog *(page 84)* | 10 |
| Goblet Squat *(page 73)* | 8 |
| Straight-Leg Deadlift *(page 77)* | 8 |
| Heel Raise *(page 78)* | 8 |
| Do 3 rounds total | |

## BASIC PROGRAM: UPPER BODY

| Chest Press *(page 63)* | 8 |
|---|:---:|
| Diamond Push-Up *(page 57)* | 4 |
| Overhead Press *(page 65)* | 6 |
| Cross-Over Push-Up *(page 58)* | 5 |
| One-Armed Row *(page 64)* | 6 each side |
| Dual Push-Up *(page 60)* | 8 |
| Bounce-Up *(page 61)* | 4 |
| Push-Up with Row *(page 62)* | 4 each side |
| Chest Fly *(page 71)* | 6 |
| Reverse Fly *(page 72)* | 6 |
| Do 3 rounds total | |

## BASIC PROGRAM: CORE

| Ab Crunch *(page 82)* | 12 |
|---|:---:|
| Plank *(page 79)* | 0:30 |
| Mason Twist *(page 81)* | 8 |
| Hip Raise/Glute Bridge *(page 85)* | 10 |
| Bird Dog *(page 84)* | 8 |
| Back Extension *(page 83)* | 8 |
| Do 4 rounds total | |

# Advanced Program

Congratulations and welcome to the Advanced BOSU Balance Trainer program! If you've done the Basic program, as we strongly urge, you should know what you're in for here. Our one solemn promise is that you're going to absolutely know you're working out when you go through this program. You won't have time to think about balance and coordination—you'll be too busy sweating! You won't have energy to worry about failing because you'll be struggling to get in one more round! The Advanced program will have you busting through plateaus and going through the stratosphere—and you'll love every agonizing minute of it!

And if the above sounds like hyperbole, we can assure you it isn't. That's why it's important to get your feet beneath you via the Basic program. If you aren't an experienced BOSUian, please, please take the time and do the Basic program. You'll thank us (and yourself) later.

A note about intensity and progression: Don't cheat yourself out of an amazing workout. Since you choose the weights and decide on how fast or hard you'll perform every movement (all with proper form, right?), it's up to you to drive yourself to get the most out of this workout. Anyone can pick light weights and sleepwalk through a routine. If you're looking to get great results you need to focus on your form and perform each exercise with the intensity that's indicative of the goal you're trying to achieve. As you progress through the program you'll get stronger and need to raise your weights in order to keep gaining strength. Choose a weight that you can perform the desired exercise with good form, but the last two reps should really make you work. If you finish a set feeling you could've done more reps, then your weight is most likely too light.

Much like the Basic program, the Advanced program is done in cycles. Follow along the list of exercises, completing an exercise for the prescribed time or reps and then moving on to the next exercise in the rotation. Once you've completed all the exercises back to back in superset fashion, that's one set. After a set you'll take a 60-second rest and then you'll continue until you've completed all 3 sets for each workout. Sounds easy, right? Well, we'll see about that!

| | MONDAY | TUESDAY | WEDNESDAY | THURSDAY | FRIDAY | SAT/SUN |
|---|---|---|---|---|---|---|
| Perform the designated workout routine on the corresponding day noted on the chart below. Rest for 1 minute between each round. | | | | | | |
| WEEK 1 | Lower Body | Core | Upper Body | Core | Lower Body | OFF |
| WEEK 2 | Upper Body | Core | Lower Body | Core | Upper Body | OFF |
| WEEK 3 | Lower Body/Core | Upper Body | OFF | Lower Body | Upper Body/Core | OFF |
| WEEK 4 | Full Body 1 | Lower Body/Core | OFF | Upper Body/Core | Full Body 2 | OFF |
| WEEK 5 | Lower Body/Core | Full Body 1 | Core | Full Body 2 | Upper Body/Core | OFF |
| WEEK 6 | Full Body 1 | Lower Body | Core | Full Body 2 | Lower Body | OFF |
| WEEK 7 | Full Body 1 | Full Body 2 | Core | Full Body 1 | Full Body 2 | OFF |

## ADVANCED PROGRAM: FULL BODY 1

| EXERCISE | REPS/TIME |
|---|:---:|
| Push-Up *(page 55)*/alternate sets with Toe-Balance Push-Up *(page 56)* | 15 reps |
| Plank *(page 79)* | 1:00 |
| Squat *(page 73)* | 15 reps |
| Mason Twist *(page 81)* | 20 reps |
| Mountain Climber *(page 86)* | 12 reps |
| Back Extension *(page 83)*/alternate sets with Reverse Fly *(page 72)* | 15/10 reps |
| Burpee *(page 87)* | 10 reps |
| Ab Crunch *(page 82)* | 20 reps |
| Diamond Push-Up *(page 57)* | 10 reps |
| Lunge *(page 76)* | 10 reps each leg |
| Front Row *(page 70)* | 12 |
| Do 3 rounds total | |

## ADVANCED PROGRAM: FULL BODY 2

| Diamond Push-Up, dome-side down *(p. 57)* | 15 reps |
|---|:---:|
| Goblet Squat *(page 73)* | 15 reps |
| Overhead Press *(page 65)*/alternate sets with Triceps Extension *(page 66)* | 15 reps |
| Bounce-Up *(page 61)* | 10 reps |
| Burpee *(page 87)* | 15 reps |
| Step-Up with Dumbbell Curl *(page 75)*/alternate sets with Triceps Kickback *(page 67)* | 10 each side |
| Plank Row *(page 80)* | 10 each side |
| Hip Raise/Glute Bridge *(page 85)* | 20 reps |
| Lunge with Dumbbell *(page 76)* | 10 reps |
| Bird Dog *(page 84)* | 20 reps |
| Front Raise *(page 69)*/alternate sets with Lateral Raise *(page 68)* | 12 |
| Do 3 rounds total | |

## ADVANCED PROGRAM: UPPER BODY

| EXERCISE | REPS/TIME |
|---|---|
| Chest Press *(page 63)* | 15 |
| Diamond Push-Up *(page 57)* | 10 |
| Overhead Press *(page 65)* | 12 |
| Cross-Over Push-Up *(page 58)* | 12 |
| One-Armed Row *(page 64)* | 12 per arm |
| Dual Push-Up *(page 60)* | 14 |
| Bounce-Up *(page 61)* | 10 |
| Push-Up with Row *(page 62)* | 12 per arm |
| Chest Fly *(page 71)* | 12 |
| Reverse Fly *(page 72)* | 10 |
| Do 3 rounds total | |

## ADVANCED PROGRAM: LOWER BODY

| | |
|---|---|
| Squat *(page 73)* | 12 |
| Step-Up with Dumbbell Curl *(page 75)* | 15 |
| Squat with Overhead Press *(page 74)* | 10 |
| Back Extension *(page 83)* | 12 |
| Lunge *(page 76)* | 10 each side |
| Lunge with Dumbbell *(page 76)* | 10 each side |
| Bird Dog *(page 84)* | 12 |
| Goblet Squat *(page 73)* | 12 |
| Straight-Leg Deadlift *(page 77)* | 10 |
| Heel Raise *(page 78)* | 12 |
| Do 3 rounds total | |

## ADVANCED PROGRAM: CORE

| | |
|---|---|
| Ab Crunch *(page 82)* | 20 |
| Plank *(page 79)* | 1:00 |
| Mason Twist *(page 81)* | 20 |
| Hip Raise/Glute Bridge *(page 85)* | 20 |
| Bird Dog *(page 84)* | 12 |
| Back Extension *(page 83)* | 12 |
| Do 4 rounds total | |

# Beyond the BOSU Balance Trainer

Is that it? Are we done? NEVER! You're never truly done when it comes to making new and better versions of yourself. We've found that as long as we remain committed to personal and physical improvement, there are always things we can do. To that end, we have some recommendations on where you can look next depending on your goals.

We're very happy that you've taken the BOSU Balance Trainer journey with us. We're even happier for you that you've gone through the program. You should have found out things about yourself, pushed your body to places you never knew you could and, more importantly, positively affected both your body and outlook on life.

And we'd love for you to continue your journey with us in other ways. Once again, it's up to you. You'll need to decide what you want next, which goal you're hoping to achieve. Are you looking to take your fitness to the next level? Perhaps consider *Ultimate Jump Rope Workouts*. Are you hoping to see your abs for the first time in years? *7 Weeks to Getting Ripped* will get you there! What about adding some solid, quality, lean muscle? *7 Weeks to 10 Pounds of Muscle* will be your guide. Maybe now that you have some base level of fitness you want to race your first triathlon, crossing it off your bucket list? *7 Weeks to Triathlon* has everything you'll need.

This book is designed to fit in with all of our books that we mentioned above. Each of the *7 Weeks to Fitness* programs has been created to be used in conjunction with the others for year-round, lifelong fitness. Choose your goals: strength, speed, endurance, flexibility, explosive power, sport-specific skills (triathlons, obstacle races, etc.), endurance or even just developing a fit, killer physique. We've created programs that are step-by-step and easy to follow. The important thing is that you get to decide your future. You have the power and we have the tools. With that combination, you can't go wrong! To make it even easier to choose, we offer all of our programs and book samples for free on www.7weekstofitness.com. Got a question? You can contact Brett and Jason there as well.

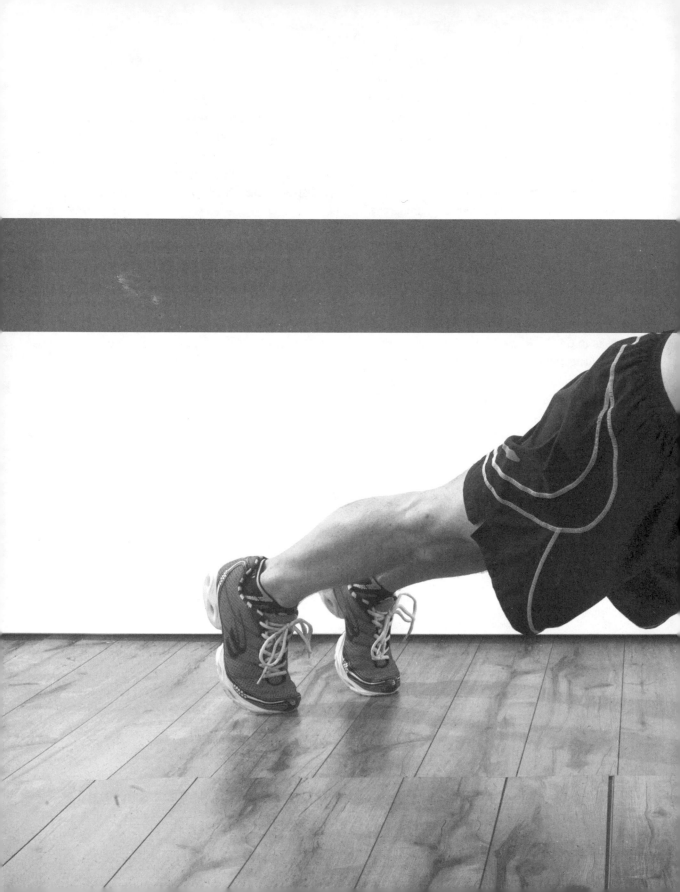

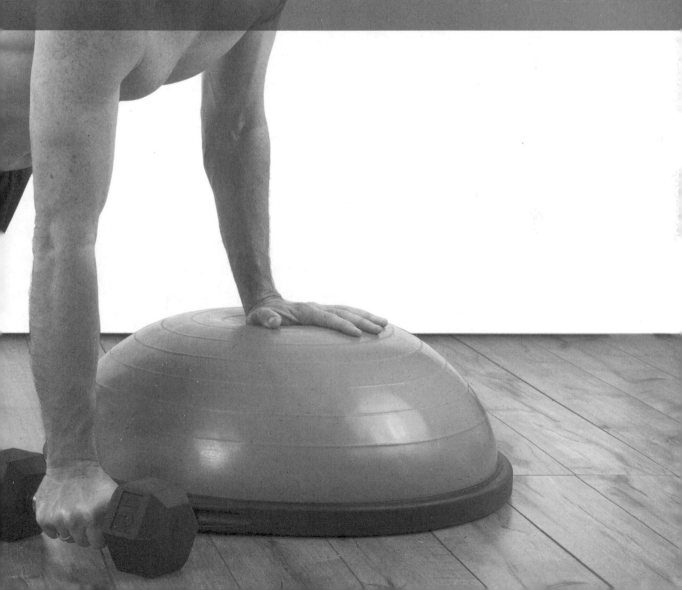

# PART III

# THE EXERCISES

# Basic Exercises

The following are the basic building blocks of the BOSU program. Master them and you'll be well on your way to mastering the BOSU Balance Trainer. The exercises are broken down into upper-body, lower-body, core and full-body movements. We highly recommend you become extremely comfortable doing all these movements before attempting any exercise in the "Extra Credit" section on page 88.

Take special note of the BOSU position listed for each exercise. The great thing about the BOSU Balance Trainer is how adaptable it is, so you can do most of these either dome-side up or dome-side down. We encourage you to experiment with each, though we'll make a strong recommendation about where to start.

*The quintessential upper-body BOSU exercise: Your upper body must react to the unstable BOSU dome and you'll soon feel the work everywhere, including your chest, shoulders, arms, back and core. Wearing a weighted vest intensifies the exercise.*

**STARTING POSITION:** Get on your hands and knees and position your hands on either side of the bull's-eye, arms fully extended. Find a placement that feels comfortable—not too wide, not too narrow. Lift your knees off the floor, tightening your core to support your whole body.

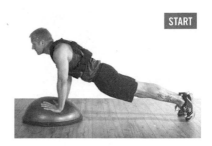

START

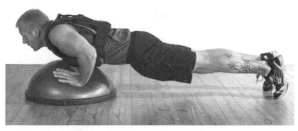

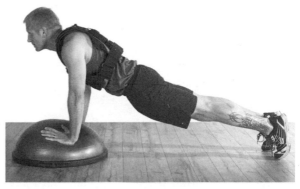

**1** Bend both elbows and lower your body until your chest touches the dome. Pause.

**2** Push yourself back to starting position.

## VARIATION

*The push-up can also be done with the dome-side down by grabbing the edges of the flat surface.*

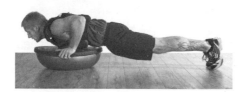

## NOTES

*Of course this is an awesome workout—core, chest and arm activation all in one movement! The great thing about the BOSU Balance Trainer is you can move your hands around and stress entirely new muscles with such a simple adjustment.*

*Increase the difficulty of the traditional push-up by forcing your core and upper body to stabilize your body while your feet wiggle. Wearing a weighted vest intensifies the work.*

**STARTING POSITION:** Get on your knees and position your toes on the dome and your hands about shoulder-width apart on the floor and under your chest. Fully extend your arms and keep your core tight.

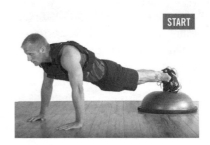
START

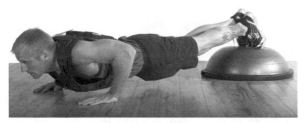

**1** Bend both elbows and lower your body until your chest nearly touches the floor. Pause.

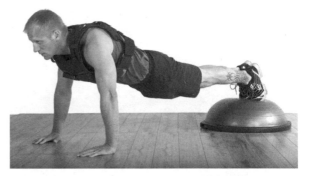

**2** Push yourself back to starting position.

**NOTES**

*This set-up changes the angle and leverage of the traditional push-up, making it more difficult. Don't be surprised if you can't do as many as you could do of the traditional push-up.*

# DIAMOND PUSH-UP

*This great triceps exercise will make you feel like you're pushing against sand, making each rep harder and more effective. Wearing a weighted vest intensifies the work.*

**STARTING POSITION:** Get on your knees and position your hands on the dome of the BOSU Balance Trainer, arms fully extended. Your thumbs and forefingers should be pressed together to form a triangle or diamond shape, with the bull's-eye in the opening between your hands. Lift your knees off the floor, tightening your core to support your whole body.

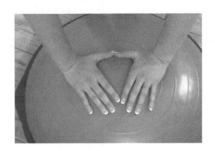

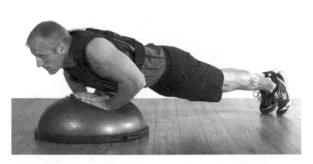

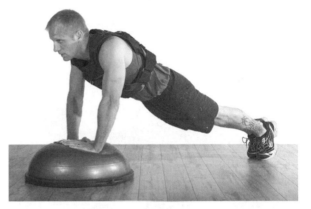

**1** Bend both elbows and lower your body until your chest touches your hands. Pause.

**2** Push yourself back to starting position.

## VARIATION

*When doing this version, be careful to be in the center of the flat surface.*

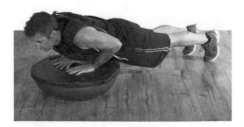

### NOTES

*This is one of the best triceps workouts there is! Don't be surprised if your arms wiggle like jelly after the first few reps.*

*When performing these push-ups, one hand will be placed on the center of the BOSU Balance Trainer, the other on the floor. Wearing a weighted vest intensifies the work.*

**STARTING POSITION:** Get on your knees and position your right hand directly on the bull's-eye, arm fully extended. Place your left hand on the floor to the left of the BOSU Balance Trainer. Your hands should be just wider than your shoulders. Lift your knees off the floor, tightening your core to support your whole body.

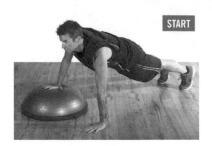

START

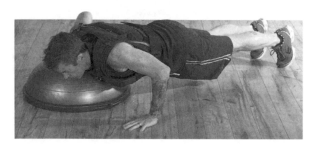

**1** Bend both elbows and lower your body until your chest is several inches off the floor. Find the point in the descent where you feel you can't descend any farther. Pause.

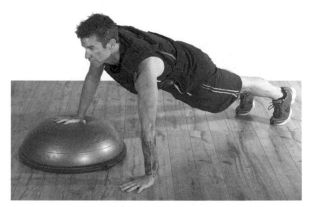

**2** Push yourself back to starting position.

**NOTES**

*To make this harder, you can start with your left hand on the floor. As you complete 1 rep, jump your right hand to the floor and your left hand to the BOSU Balance Trainer. This creates an explosive movement.*

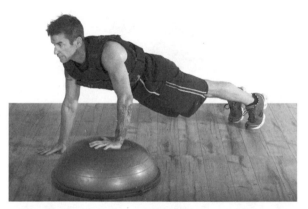

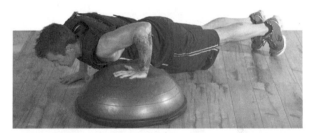

**3** Place your left hand next to your right on top of the dome and reposition your right hand on the floor to the left of the BOSU Balance Trainer.

If you're unsteady, place your knees on the floor during the cross-over transition.

**4** Lower down and then push yourself back up to starting position. That's 1 rep.

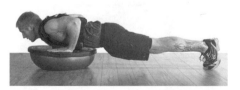

*You'll need two BOSU Balance Trainers for this one. Wearing a weighted vest intensifies the work.*

**STARTING POSITION:** Get on your knees and position each hand on a bull's-eye, arms fully extended. The BOSU position should make your hands just wider than your shoulders; adjust if needed. Lift your knees off the floor, tightening your core to support your whole body.

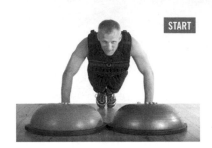

START

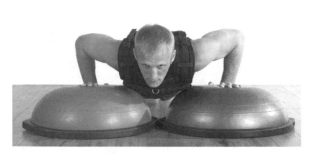

**1** Bend both elbows and lower your body until your chest touches the BOSU. Pause.

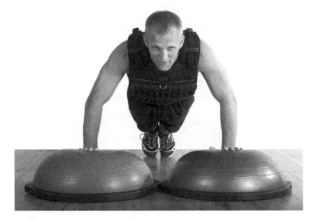

**2** Push yourself back to starting position.

**VARIATION**

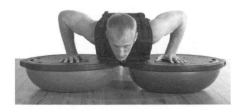

**NOTES**

*Because of the size of the BOSU Balance Trainers, with the dome-side-up version your hand position will most likely be wider than normal, emphasizing your chest instead of your arms. With the dome-side down, you can play with different hand positions all over the bases to maximize the workout for your arms, chest and even shoulders. The instability will also cause your core to work overtime to keep your back straight and flat.*

*This is an explosive push-up variant that will be sure to leave you dripping with sweat. Like Bounce-Ups? Then you'll love Bounce Around the Clock on page 97. Although the BOSU Balance Trainer serves as a weight, wearing a weighted vest intensifies the work.*

**STARTING POSITION:** Get on your knees and grasp the sides of the flat surface, arms fully extended. Lift your knees off the floor, tightening your core to support your whole body.

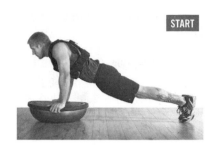

START

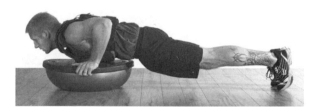

**1** Bend both elbows and lower your body until your chest touches the BOSU Balance Trainer. Pause.

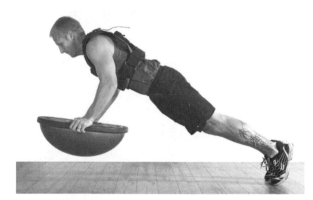

**2** Explode up, pushing yourself back toward the starting position. You'll need to use enough force to lift the BOSU Balance Trainer off the floor.

**3** Brace yourself and land with your elbows slightly bent to cushion against the impact, then lower your body until your chest touches the BOSU Balance Trainer.

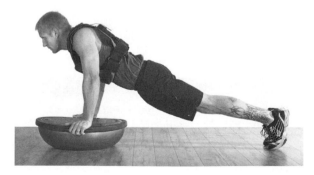

**NOTES**

*The shock absorber/trampoline effect of the dome makes the impact a bit less harsh than doing a standard plyometric push-up. Also, keeping your hands on the BOSU Balance Trainer forces you to use a variety of core and upper-body muscles to keep it in place while promoting muscular symmetry as your chest and arms need to produce equal amounts of explosive power to keep your motion straight up.*

*Adding one-arm rows to the Push-Up (page 55) activates the biceps more.*

**STARTING POSITION:** Get on your knees and place your right hand directly on the bull's-eye, with your right arm fully extended. Place your left hand on the handle of a dumbbell resting flat on the floor below your shoulder. Assume a three-point plank position with your feet wider than your shoulders and your back flat.

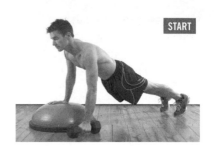

START

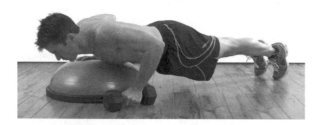

**1** Keeping your back flat and core engaged, bend both elbows and lower your chest toward the floor. Pause when your chest touches the dome.

**2** Push yourself back to starting position.

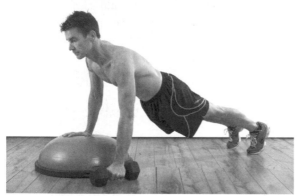

**3** When you're in top position, bend your left elbow and pull the dumbbell to your torso, pointing your elbow directly at the ceiling. Pause.

Return the dumbbell to starting position. That's 1 rep.

Repeat, then switch hands.

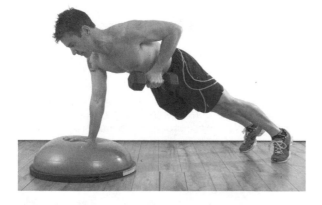

**NOTES**

*It's amazing how well this works your core. Keep the movement strict and tight and you'll know you're working it hard. It also works your upper back, chest and both the biceps and triceps all in one movement.*

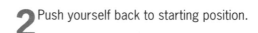

# DUMBBELL CHEST PRESS

*The classic dumbbell bench press is even more effective on the BOSU Balance Trainer. Now you're working your core, legs and upper body all at the same time.*

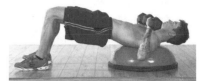

START

**STARTING POSITION:** Lie with your upper back supported on the bull's-eye, knees bent and feet firmly planted on the floor slightly wider than your shoulders. Grasp a dumbbell with each hand and curl the weights into position at chest level, with your thumbs parallel with your chest. Engage your core, squeeze your glutes together and press your hips toward the ceiling to form a bridge position, with your torso parallel to the floor and flat from chest to knees.

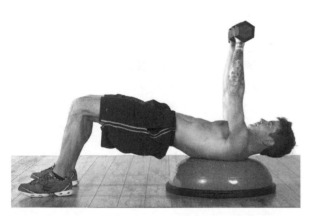

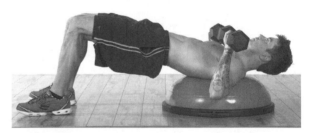

**1** Pushing from your chest, slowly extend your arms fully to raise the weights up toward the ceiling. Pause.

**2** Slowly lower the weights to starting position.

---

**NOTES**

*Simple yet extremely effective, the bench press is a natural complement to push-ups as both are fantastic upper-body strength-building exercises. By performing these on the BOSU Balance Trainer, the additional hip raise and bridge movement make this a compound exercise responsible for activating nearly your whole body.*

*This variant of a traditional back exercise becomes a complete core workout as well.*

**STARTING POSITION:** Get on your knees and place your right knee on the bull's-eye. Extend your left leg straight out behind you and place your toe on the floor for balance. Place your right hand on the floor directly below your shoulder, arm fully extended; your back should form a flat tabletop position. Grasp a weight in your right hand.

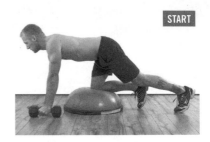

START

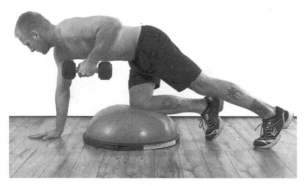

**1** Squeezing your left lat (back) muscle, bend your elbow to pull the weight into your torso. Pause.

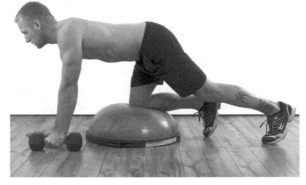

**2** Slowly lower the weight to starting position.

**NOTES**

*Focus on squeezing your back at the top and lowering the weights slowly. The instability of performing this move on the BOSU Balance Trainer activates your core and hips, making it a compound movement.*

# OVERHEAD PRESS

*One of the "Power Four" exercises along with squat, chest press and deadlift to build power and strength, this exercise can be performed with a medicine ball, dumbbells or a weighted bar. Keep your knees slightly bent in an athletic position and don't let them bow in during the exercise. Keep your core engaged throughout the entire movement to keep your spine in a natural position.*

**STARTING POSITION:** Using an overhand grip, grasp the weighted bar with hands a little wider than your shoulders and raise it until it's even with your collarbone. Stand on the dome with each foot on either side of the center. Find a stable position, turning your toes outward a few degrees in order to maintain your balance.

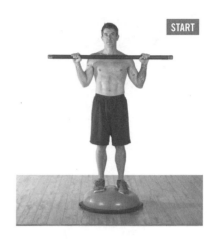
START

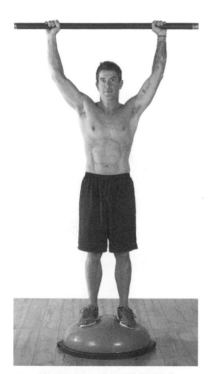

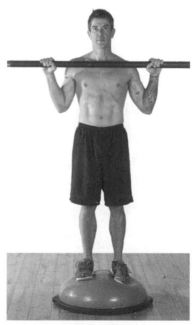

**1** Exhale and extend your arms directly overhead, pressing the weight up until your arms are fully extended. Pause.

**2** Slowly, in a controlled manner, lower the bar back down to starting position.

**VARIATION: DUMBBELLS**

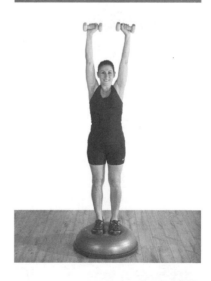

*This triceps-isolation exercise stimulates full-body activation when performed on the BOSU Balance Trainer.*

**STARTING POSITION:** Stand with both feet on the dome, with arms grasping dumbbells over and behind your head, elbows raised into a position nearly in line with your ears and bent about 90 degrees.

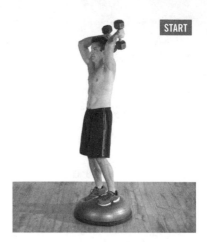

START

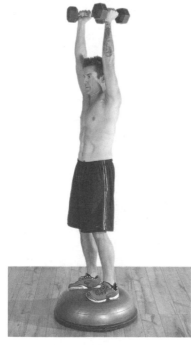

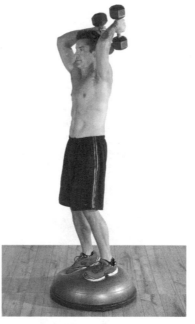

**1** Press the weights forward and upward toward the ceiling by extending your elbows. Pause.

**2** Return to starting position.

**NOTES**

*You should feel this only in your triceps. If you feel stress or pressure on your elbows, switch to lighter weights.*

# TRICEPS KICKBACK

*Another great triceps-isolation exercise, this one engages the core more significantly.*

**STARTING POSITION:** Start with your right knee on the dome and your left hand supporting your weight either on the ground or the edge of the BOSU Balance Trainer. Extend your left leg behind you with both toes on the ground for balance. Grasp the dumbbell with your right hand and raise it to your right hip.

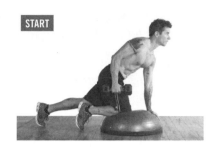

**START**

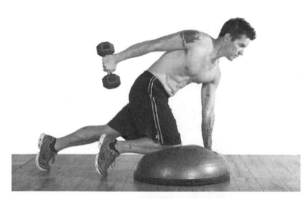

**1** Extend your elbow and press the dumbbell directly behind you by engaging your triceps. Don't rotate your shoulder; try to limit rotation of your torso. Your triceps should be doing all the work! Pause.

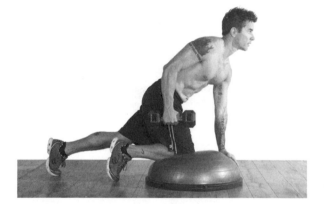

**2** Return to the starting position.

Finish the desired reps and repeat on the opposite side.

**NOTES**

*The more you position your torso over the BOSU Balance Trainer, the more your core is engaged. Play with positions to find what works for you and over time challenges your balance more to get a better workout.*

*This exercise works the outer shoulders, but adding the BOSU Balance Trainer forces you to engage your core for a more full-body workout.*

**STARTING POSITION:** Stand on the dome with your feet about shoulder-width apart and knees slightly bent. Hold the dumbbells at your sides with your palms facing your upper legs.

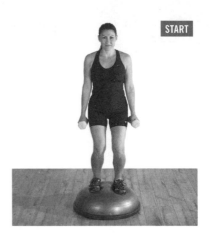

START

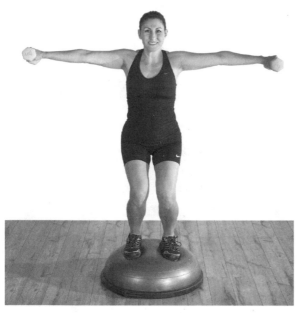

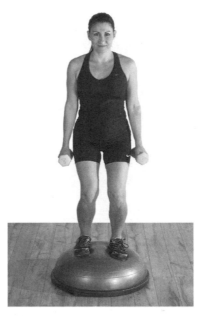

**1** Keeping your arms fully extended, slowly raise the dumbbells in an arc up to shoulder height. Pause.

**2** Slowly return to starting position.

**NOTES**

*This exercise is great for your deltoids, a controlled and isolated exercise with a full range of motion along a singular plane.*

*Strengthen and sculpt your shoulders while engaging your core to maintain balance and proper posture. Because you're using small stabilizing muscles in your shoulders, be sure to use light weights. If you have any pain or limited range of motion, you may need to drop down in weight or practice the move using your bare hands.*

**STARTING POSITION:** Stand on the dome with your feet about shoulder-width apart and knees slightly bent. Hold the dumbbells with both palms facing your body, arms fully extended and weights at the tops of your thighs.

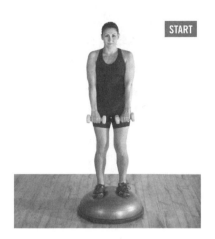

START

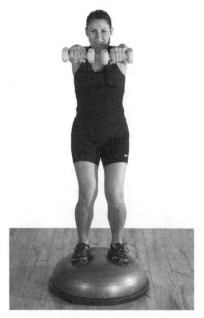

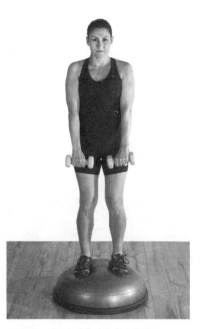

**1** Keeping your arms fully extended, raise the dumbbells slowly in a forward arc directly in front of your torso, stopping when they reach shoulder height. Pause.

**2** In a slow and controlled motion, return to starting position.

**NOTES**

*Stabilizing your body on the BOSU Balance Trainer becomes a little more difficult when you extend those weights directly out in front of you. Remember to keep your core tight and back straight to maintain proper posture.*

**PRIMARY MUSCLES: DELTOIDS, TRAPEZIUS**
**SECONDARY MUSCLES: BICEPS, CORE**

*The weights work your upper back and arms, the chest fly performed on the BOSU Balance Trainer forces you to maintain proper posture and balance to complete the move.*

**STARTING POSITION:** Stand on the dome with your feet approximately shoulder-width apart and knees slightly bent. Grasp the dumbbells in both hands with your palms facing your body. Extend your arms fully in front of your legs and bend at the waist about 45–60 degrees.

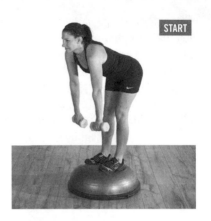

START

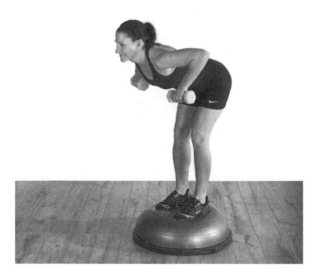

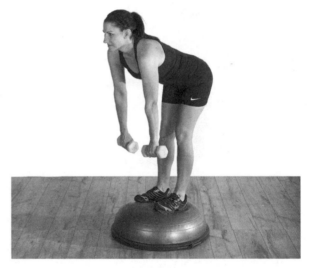

**1** Using your biceps and the large muscles in your upper back, bend your elbows and pull the dumbbells to your sides just below your chest. Pause.

**2** Slowly return to starting position.

**NOTES**

*This exercise is meant to primarily use your back muscles; your arms are just supporting the effort. If you don't feel this in your upper back, focus on pulling your shoulder blades together in order to raise your elbows directly to the ceiling. With proper upper back activation, you may find that you can lift heavier weights.*

*A great exercise to target the pectoral muscles, the chest fly performed on the BOSU Balance Trainer allows you to utilize your core, hips and upper legs to maintain proper posture.*

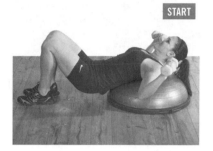

START

**STARTING POSITION:** Lying on the dome, position your shoulder blades so they're approximately on either side of the bull's-eye. Grasp a dumbbell in each hand with an overhand grip, bend both elbows approximately 90 degrees, and position your arms in line with your torso. The weights should be slightly above shoulder height with your inner arms and palms facing the ceiling. Raise your buttocks off the ground for the entire movement; keep your core tight in order to stabilize your back.

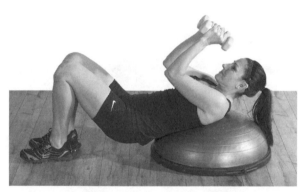

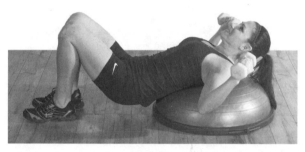

**1** Keeping your elbows bent and your wrists in a locked position, engage your pectoral muscles to lift the weights—slowly swing them in an arc together directly over your sternum. Pause when your palms are facing each other and the weights are gently touching. Squeeze your chest together during the movement and especially when the weights are above your torso. Pause.

**2** Slowly return to starting position.

### VARIATION

*This can also be done with wrist weights.*

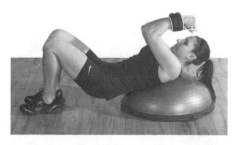

### NOTES

*Chest flys are very effective at targeting your pecs and sculpting your chest muscles but should be done with a lighter weight as you'll also be placing some of the burden on stabilizing muscles in your shoulders.*

*Initially, this will feel like a strange movement, but stick with it and you'll find it to be an important part of developing upper-body strength.*

**STARTING POSITION:** Lie face-down on top of the dome with the bull's-eye centered on your torso slightly below your chest. Extend your legs and place your toes on the floor for balance. Grasp dumbbells in each hand with an overhand grip and place them on the floor, your arms nearly extended out on both sides of your shoulders. Squeeze your glutes to help brace your core. *Note:* Your elbows should be bent slightly, about 140–160 degrees relative to your upper arm.

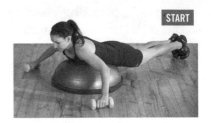

START

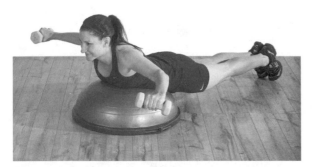

**1** Keeping your back straight and arms flat (don't rotate your forearms relative to your upper arms), lift the weights straight up off the floor using the large muscles of your upper back by squeezing your shoulder blades together. Pause at the top.

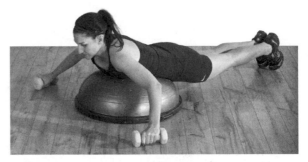

**2** Lower slowly back to starting position.

## VARIATION

*This can also be done with wrist weights.*

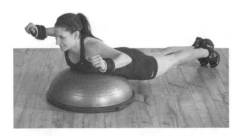

## NOTES

*Do you want a strong chest? Then you need to work the muscles of your upper back equally as much as you work your pecs. Performing this exercise on the BOSU Balance Trainer also adds some additional core work too; did you notice the plank position you're in?*

*The squat is the cornerstone of any lower-body workout. The weighted goblet variant makes the classic squat even more effective. As with most BOSU Balance Trainer exercises, this can be done dome-side down or dome-side up. Decide on the version that you find most comfortable to start and work your way to the other.*

**STARTING POSITION:** Stand on the dome with your feet on either side of the bull's-eye. Hold a dumbbell with both hands at about chest level, just below your chin. Find a stable position, turning your toes outward a few degrees in order to allow your knees to track straight up and down throughout the movement. Engage your core and rotate your hips backward slightly to initiate the movement.

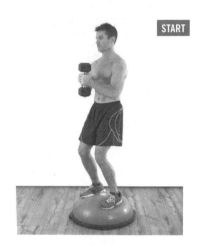

START

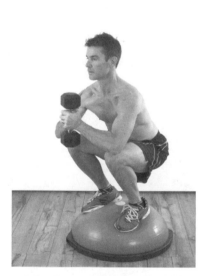

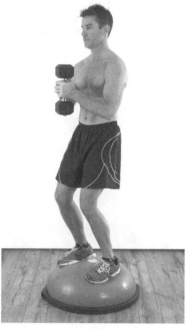

**VARIATIONS**

*This can also be done without a weight and with the dome-side down.*

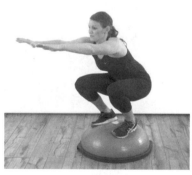

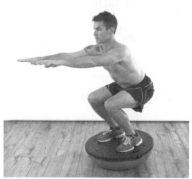

**1** Bend your knees and lower your body until your butt drops to just beyond parallel. Keep your knees over your toes; do not lean forward. Pause.

**2** Push up with your legs, returning to starting position.

*This simple full-body movement incorporates the multi-joint, multi-muscle effectiveness of a squat and couples it with the upper-body strength-building overhead press.*

**STARTING POSITION:** Stand on the dome with your feet on either side of the bull's-eye. Find a stable position. Grasp a dumbbell in each hand and raise them just above shoulder height. Engage your core to maintain your balance.

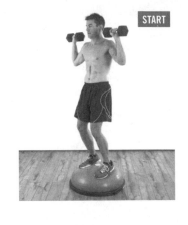

**START**

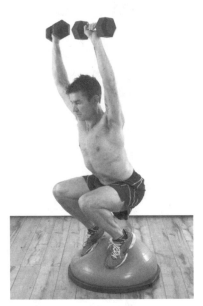

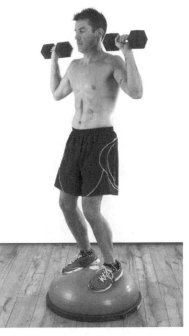

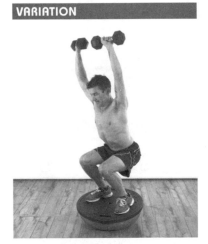

**VARIATION**

**1** Bend your knees and lower your body until your butt drops to just beyond parallel. Keep your knees over your toes; do not lean forward. At the same time, straighten your elbows and extend your arms directly overhead. Pause.

**2** Push up with your legs and lower the dumbbells, returning to starting position.

**NOTES**

*For maximum effectiveness, make sure you engage your core to stabilize and really squeeze your abs and glutes as you press the weights straight up overhead. This move will really test your balance.*

*This move is designed to strengthen your biceps while activating your core to maintain your posture. The description seems pretty easy, but this is a compound move requiring balance and coordination—performing this properly on the BOSU Balance Trainer makes sure to activate your core and lower body while your arms are getting a great workout.*

**STARTING POSITION:** With the BOSU Balance Trainer approximately half a stride's length in front of you, stand upright with a dumbbell in each hand, arms fully extended at your sides. Step on the bull's-eye one foot at a time.

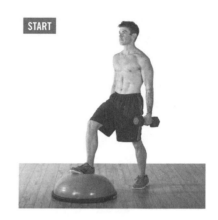
START

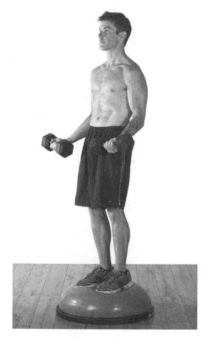

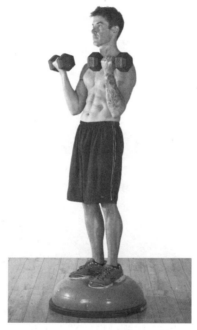

**1** Bring your elbows in toward your sides and rotate your hands so that your palms face upward.

**2** Contracting your abs to keep your spine straight and keeping your upper arms next to your torso, slowly raise the weights toward your shoulders.

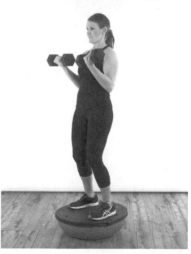
VARIATION

*Sometimes called a "split squat," this is an unbelievably effective quadriceps exercise. Bonus BOSU points are awarded to the fact that your glutes will also feel it.*

**STARTING POSITION:** With the BOSU Balance Trainer approximately half a stride's length in front of you, stand upright with a dumbbell in each hand, arms fully extended at your sides.

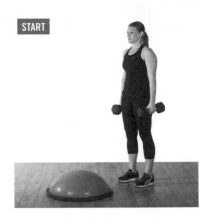

START

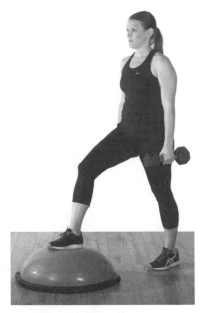

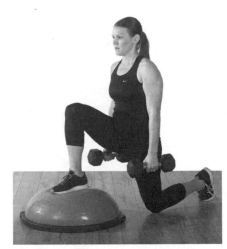

**1** Place your right toes directly in the middle of the bull's-eye with your right knee bent slightly. Support your weight on your left leg, with most of it through your heel, not your toes.

**2** Bend your right leg and begin to descend your right knee and glutes toward the floor. Gently touch your left knee to the ground and pause.

Push through your right heel and return to starting position.

Switch sides.

**NOTES**

*Master this move on the ground before you even think of sliding a BOSU Balance Trainer into position and you'll reap the benefits by performing it correctly.*

*Working your lower back, glutes and hamstrings, the straight-leg deadlift on the BOSU Balance Trainer is an excellent way to keep your focus on your form—otherwise you'll lose your balance!*

**STARTING POSITION:** Holding dumbbells in both hands, stand on the apex of the dome with both feet on opposite sides of the bull's-eye. Fully extend your arms with your palms facing your upper thighs.

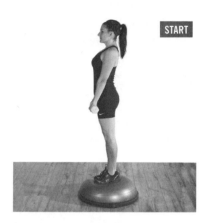

START

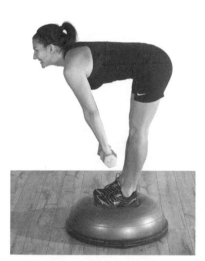

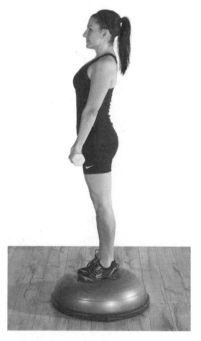

**1** Rotate your hips backward slightly and bend at your waist, keeping your arms fully extended and the weights as close as possible to your legs. Keep your back flat through the movement and continue bending until your back is parallel to the floor. Pause.

**2** Squeeze your glutes, drive through your heels and use your hamstrings and lower back to raise you back to starting position.

**NOTES**

*A fantastic example of a multi-joint, multi-muscle exercise, the straight-leg deadlift is not only great for developing a stronger lower back and hamstrings, it's also responsible for developing a more shapely posterior.*

*On a flat surface, a heel raise is a very good exercise to strengthen and elongate your calf muscles. When performed with weights on a BOSU Balance Trainer, it becomes even more effective at developing coordination, balance and activating supporting muscles all over your body.*

**STARTING POSITION:** Stand directly on the bull's-eye with both feet together, holding a dumbbell in each hand with arms extended and palms facing your hips. Engage your core to keep your back straight.

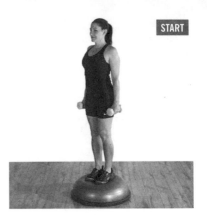

START

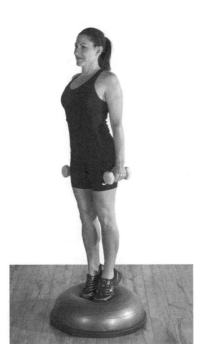

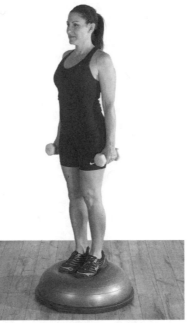

**1** Press through your toes to raise your heels up and off the dome. Pause when your feet are fully extended and maintain your balance for 3–5 seconds.

**2** Slowly return to starting position.

**NOTES**

*At first this may feel a bit awkward, but after a few reps you should get the hang of it. After a few more reps your calves should be burning!*

*You can do this complete core movement with either your hands, feet or forearms on the BOSU Balance Trainer. Wearing a weighted vest intensifies the work.*

**THE POSITION:** Get on your knees and put your hands on the dome under your chest on both sides of the bull's-eye. Lift your knees off the floor. Only your toes and hands should be supporting your full weight. Engage your core, keeping a straight line from your heels to head. Hold this position for the duration of the exercise.

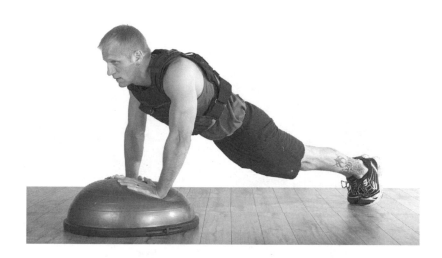

## NOTES

*The instability of the BOSU Balance Trainer forces your obliques into action to keep your back flat and works your glutes and hips much more than a plank on the flat ground does to keep your lower body straight. Switch up between dome-side up and down to target your upper and lower abs differently.*

## VARIATION

*The plank can also be done with the dome-side down by grabbing the edges of the flat surface.*

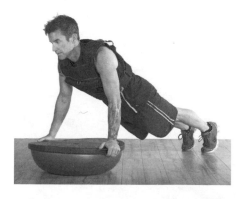

*Think the plank was hard? Add some one-arm rows to the mix and you'll be working up a sweat before you can get through one rep!*

**STARTING POSITION:** Get on your knees and place your right hand directly on the bull's-eye, right arm fully extended. Hold a dumbbell in your left hand. Lift your knees off the floor and extend your legs behind you with your feet wider than your shoulders. Keep your back flat and core engaged throughout the exercise.

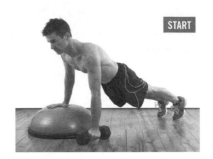

START

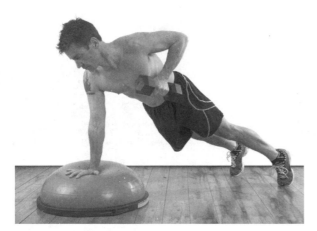

**1** Bend your left elbow and pull the dumbbell to your torso, pointing your elbow directly at the ceiling. Pause.

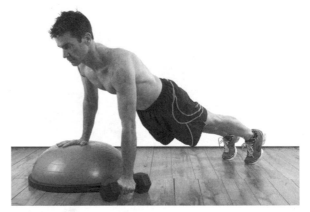

**2** Return the dumbbell to starting position. Complete half the required reps with your left hand rowing the weight, then switch hands.

**NOTES**

*Adding rows brings a whole new dimension to this classic exercise. Suddenly it's a compound move and your upper body gets in on the fun while increasing the instability that causes your core to work even more. That's a win-win in our book!*

*This complete, dynamic core movement targets your core and obliques and has a massive impact as you progress in weights used.*

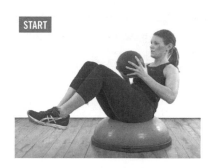

START

**STARTING POSITION:** Sit comfortably in the middle of the dome and either hold a weight with both hands or clasp your hands together. Using your core, lift your legs off the ground, knees bent slightly. Keep your heels approximately 3–6 inches off the ground for the duration. You should be in somewhat of a "V" position, albeit with your knees bent.

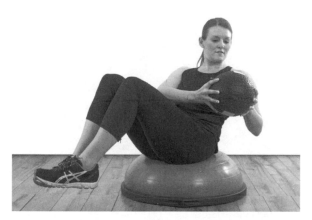

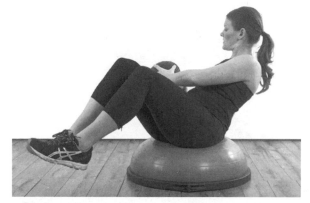

**1** Twist your torso to one side, bringing your hands (and the weight) with your torso.

**2** Smoothly twist your torso through the center and to the other side, bringing your hands (and the weight) with you.

**NOTES**

*Sometimes we call this the core shredder. It's one of those "Hey, this is easy...wait a minute...woah, I'm pooped" exercises that works your abs, lower back and hips by getting in the "V" position, and your obliques by completing the twisting motion. For optimum core strength and reduced risk of lower back pain, perform the entire move in a slow and controlled manner.*

*This standard abdominal crunch on the BOSU Balance Trainer activates even more of your core muscles due to the instability of the dome.*

**STARTING POSITION:** Sit on the dome slightly forward of the apex, lean backward, engage your core to keep your back straight and plant your feet on the ground.

***NOTE:*** If the feet-up version is too difficult at first, start with your feet on the floor (see the weighted variation below).

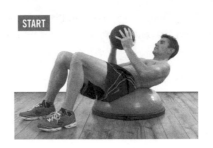

START

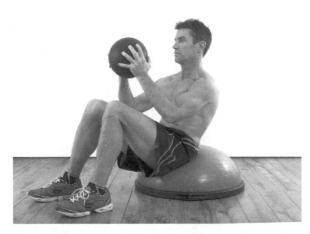

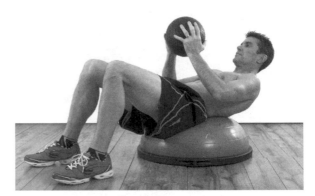

**1** Using your abs, pull your chest toward your knees in a smooth, non-jerking motion. Pause at the top and hold this position with abs contracted for 1–3 seconds.

**2** Keeping your feet on the ground, slowly return to starting position.

**VARIATION**

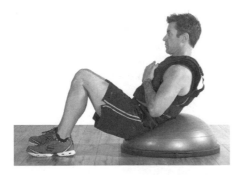

**NOTES**

*The simplest of all ab exercises, the additional instability activates your entire trunk, including obliques, hip flexors and upper legs. Focus on the isometric contraction at the top of the crunch. Pretty simple and straightforward: This. Strengthens. Abs. Actually, it helps to work your entire core, forcing your lower back to stabilize your spine when straightening and your hips when contracting.*

# BACK EXTENSION

*This great core strengthener should be the focal point of everyone with lower back issues. Wearing ankle and/or wrist weights intensifies the work.*

**STARTING POSITION:** Lie down with your belly button on the bull's-eye, hands extended in front of you. Engage your core.

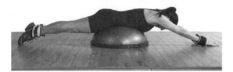

**1** Pulling through your glutes and lower back, lift your head, hands and feet off the ground. Pause.

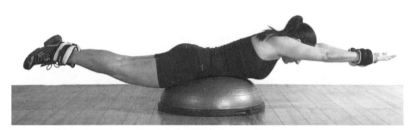

**2** In a slow and controlled manner, return to starting position, focusing on keeping your core tight and arms and legs fully extended. Do not arch or sag your body over the BOSU Balance Trainer.

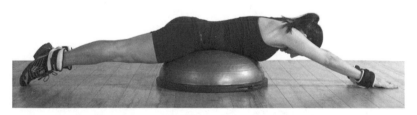

## NOTES

*Most of us have some form of soreness from sitting too much in the car or at a desk all day at work. This move will help stretch and strengthen your lower back, and stabilize your spine for better front and back core strength. If you spend any time working on your abs, you need to invest an equal amount of time performing exercises like this that strengthen your back. Period.*

*This great glute exercise also targets the lower back and can also help with shoulder stability and mobility. Wearing ankle and/or wrist weights intensifies the work.*

**STARTING POSITION:** Get on your hands and knees and place both knees directly under each hip, beside each other on the apex of the BOSU Balance Trainer. Your hands should be on the floor with arms fully extended. Keep your back flat and core engaged throughout the exercise.

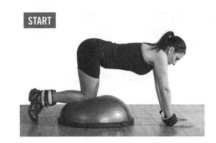
START

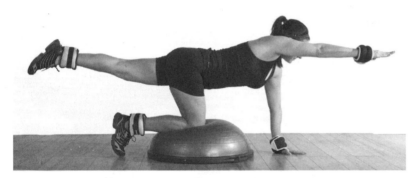

**1** Using your glutes, fully extend your left leg through your heel and lift it upward. Simultaneously raise your extended right arm forward. Pause at the top.

Lower your arm and leg toward starting position but don't touch the ground. As you near the start, pause.

Complete half of your reps with your right knee on the dome, then switch legs.

**NOTES**

*Focus on the contraction at the top; squeeze the glutes and lower back. Maintaining your balance point on the BOSU Balance Trainer with your knee can be difficult and taxing on your core, so take it slowly at first and then take it even more slowly once you get the hang of it to increase the core work.*

# HIP RAISE/GLUTE BRIDGE

*An often-overlooked exercise (maybe because it's just not all that sexy?), this is the best glutes and hip exercise for developing flexibility and strength.*

**STARTING POSITION:** Lie on the ground with your feet on the bull's-eye or flat base and your knees bent. Balance a weight on your hips, keeping it in place with your hands. Engage your core, and squeeze your glutes together.

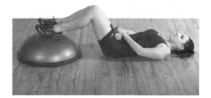

START

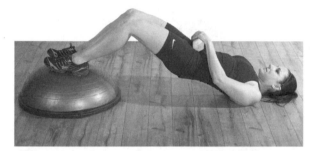

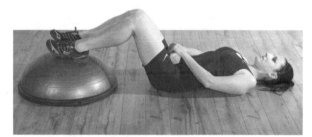

**1** Pushing through your heels, raise your hips upward until fully extended. Your body should form a straight line from sternum to knees; your upper back, head and shoulders should remain on the ground along with your arms and hands. Pause.

**2** Return to starting position.

## ADVANCED VARIATION

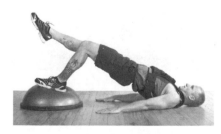

To work your core even more, raise one leg and point your toe at the top of the movement; your body should form a straight line from your sternum to your toe. Remember to switch sides.

### NOTES

*Any athlete knows that speed comes from your glutes and this has always been a staple when working out for sports. Additionally, most people actually have weak glutes and core, leading to lower back pain. Do this and you'll soon see those aches and pains go away. As triathletes, we're come to realize that hip flexibility, strength, durability and endurance are incredibly important to keep pushing hard on the bike and maintaining proper form and turnover during the run.*

*A sweat inducer in mere seconds, this exercise will get your heart pumping, your metabolism cranked and your entire body worked in a short time. Strapping on ankle weights intensifies the work your lower body has to do.*

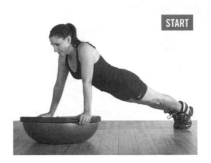

START

**STARTING POSITION:** Get on your knees and grasp the edges of the flat surface, arms fully extended. Pick up your knees off the floor. Only your toes and hands should be making contact. Engage your core, keeping a straight line from your heels to head.

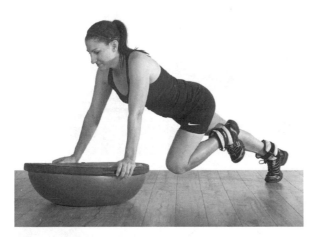

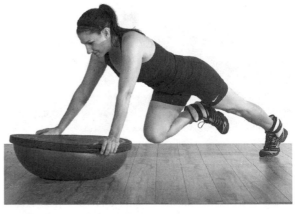

**1** As quickly as you can, bring your left knee toward your chest.

**2** Equally quickly, return your left leg to starting position. As your left toes touch the ground, bring your right knee to your chest.

Continue switching legs.

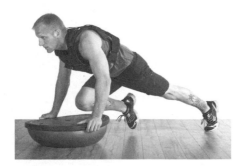

**NOTES**

*Mountain climbers are second only to burpees in their ability to get your heart pumping and metabolism revving.*

*There's no walking through this one. You'll need to focus because this is a killer workout. Your entire body will be screaming. It's simple math: Burpees + BOSU Balance Trainer = an amazing, butt-kicking exercise sure to leave you sweating and asking for more! Strapping on weights (wrist, ankle or both) intensifies the work you do.*

**STARTING POSITION:** Stand approximately half a body's length behind the BOSU Balance Trainer.

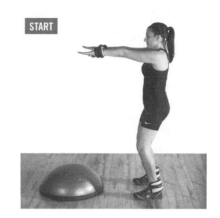

**START**

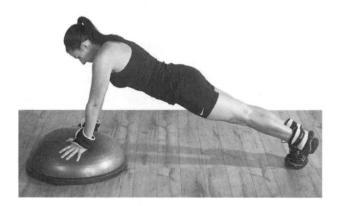

**1** Smoothly jump your feet backward, landing softly on your toes. Simultaneously drop your upper body toward the BOSU Balance Trainer, softly landing your hands on either side of the bull's-eye.

**2** Using your arms and chest, push your upper body away from the BOSU Balance Trainer while bending at the waist and jumping your feet forward, back under your body. Land with your knees slightly bent in an athletic position, arms extended. That's 1 rep.

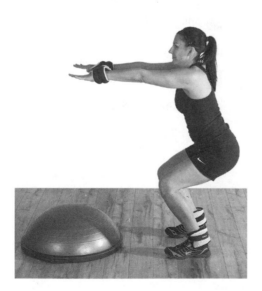

### NOTES

*Gasping for breath in maybe 5 reps. Sweating like crazy in 10. Hoping the pain will stop by 15. Giving up and just doing it at 20. Burpees are challenging yet fun and require a lot of focus to perform properly.*

# Extra Credit

We like to call these exercises "Extra Credit" because they're not included in the Basic or Advanced workouts—that is, until you add them in! In the case of the Plyometric Skater Hops and One-Legged Squats, you can swap them out for their counterpart exercise in the program to make the Basic and Advanced programs even more challenging. We strongly suggest that you complete both of the programs based on the original exercises before you swap these advanced moves in so you can develop the strength, flexibility, agility and mental acuity to perform them properly. As with all the other earlier exercises, we implore you to practice these extreme moves on a flat, stable surface and perfect your form before you attempt them on the BOSU Balance Trainer.

*This wonderful hamstring workout also develops the glutes and works on balance.*

**STARTING POSITION:** Holding a dumbbell in each hand at your sides, stand with both feet on either side of the bull's-eye. Find a stable position. Engage your core.

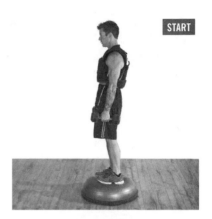

START

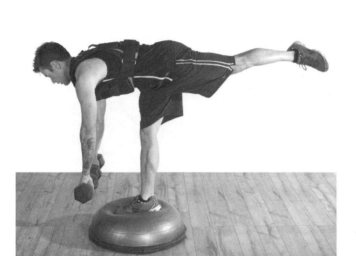

**1** Lift your left foot, fully extend your right leg and bend at the waist. Simultaneously lower your upper body and raise your left leg behind you until your entire backside, all the way from your left heel to your head, forms one straight line. Pause.

Pull through your right hamstring and glutes to return to starting position.

Repeat, then switch sides.

**NOTES**

*This a great hamstring and glute workout that can also get you a deep stretch in the hamstring. Take your time with it; don't rush through the movement. When done properly, this is actually an extremely graceful move. When performed improperly, you may end up looking like a drunk flamingo bobbing for imaginary minnows. Perfect this move on flat ground before even thinking about stepping onto a BOSU Balance Trainer or picking up a dumbbell.*

*Get ready to crank up your metabolism as this works your entire lower body and core while really getting the ol' heart a-pumping. Throughout the entire movement, keep your shoulders and pelvis level and parallel to the floor—don't lean your body forward or to the side during the downward motion, if only a tiny little bit as you initiate the explosive upward motion.*

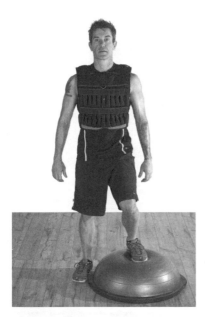

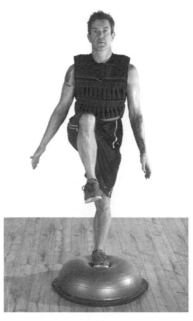

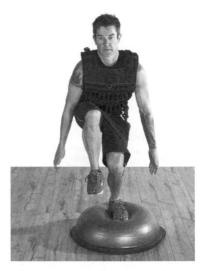

**STARTING POSITION:** Stand with your left foot directly on the bull's-eye and your right foot on the floor beside the BOSU Balance Trainer. Find a stable position and engage your core. Your arms should hang along your sides. Wearing a weighted vest intensifies the work.

**1** Shifting your weight onto your left foot and balancing on the apex of the dome, lift your right foot off the floor and bend your knee 90 degrees (about hip level). In order to keep your balance, you may tap the toes of your elevated leg to the ground for balance. As your balance and stability improve, work toward raising the knee of your "up" leg toward your chest.

**2** Bend your left knee, rotate your hips back slightly and sink straight down into a squat position (page "Goblet Squat" on page 73). Keep your left shin vertical and don't let your knee buckle to the right or left; place your right foot down and re-start if you lose your balance. *Note:* You'll most likely not be able to perform a full squat at first; descend as far as you can while maintaining good form. You should be able to go deeper as you progress in your training.

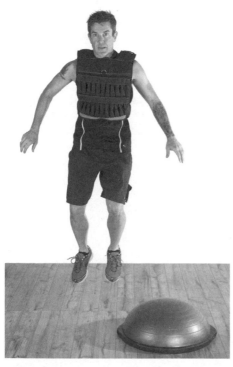

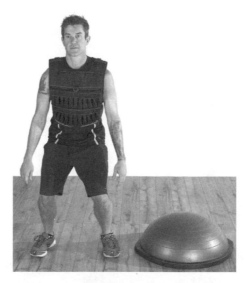

**3** Swing both arms forward and in one explosive move straighten your left leg and hop directly to your right, landing with your right foot first and then your left. Align both feet parallel to each other, with knees slightly bent to absorb the impact of landing.

**4** Stand up and return to starting position.

Repeat, then switch sides.

**NOTES**

*Seriously, get ready to feel the burn with this one! Even though you're not stabilizing on one leg for long periods of time, the plyometric motion from an unbalanced state is sure to make your quads quiver! Take it slowly. Start with just a partial squat with the leg on the BOSU Balance Trainer and perform small hops until you get the hang of it. Once you do, have a blast (while keeping good form, of course).*

*It takes some persistence and coordination to get the hang of this explosive and complete lower-body movement but it's well worth it. Wearing a weighted vest intensifies the work.*

**STARTING POSITION:** With the BOSU Balance Trainer approximately a stride's length in front of you, stand upright with your hands along your sides.

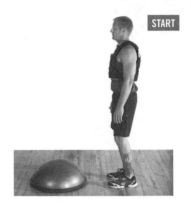
START

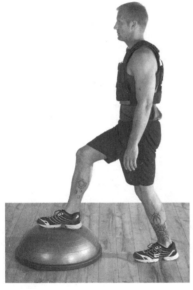

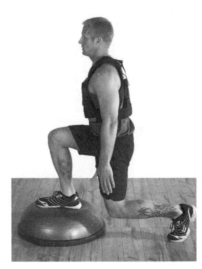

**1** Keeping your left leg in place, stride forward with your right leg, bending your right knee slightly. Land your right mid-foot directly on the bull's-eye, keeping your right knee behind your toes.

**2** Continue the stride's natural descent until your left knee almost touches the ground.

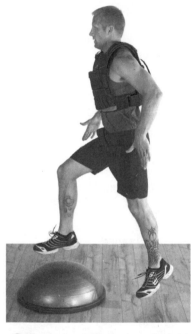

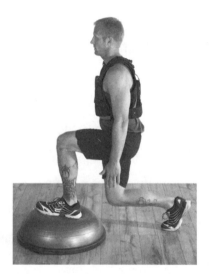

**3** Explode up through your right heel and mid-foot and switch leg positions at the peak of your jump. You should use enough force to leave the ground with both feet.

**4** Land your left mid-foot directly on the bull's-eye, aiming to keep your left knee behind your toes.

Continue the stride's natural descent until your right knee almost touches the ground.

**NOTES**

*The mid-air swap is commonly referred to as a "linear reactive," but whatever you call it, this is a complicated exercise that you need to perfect with good form on flat ground first. Be extremely careful to not let either your front knee or back knee bow inward as this can cause injury. The shin of your front leg should be perpendicular to the floor while your back leg should be balanced on your toe with the shin parallel to the ground.*

# Extreme Exercises

If you've ever picked up any of our 7 Weeks books (see www.7weekstofitness.com for a complete list of titles), this is about the point where you'll be thinking: "OK, guys, I've completed the Basic and Advanced programs and am looking for that little something extra!" Well, we try not to disappoint and always like to provide some challenging and exciting additional exercises that are a bit on the "extreme" side. The ones here are no exception. These aren't found in the Basic or Advanced programs, so it's up to you to learn how to perform each of them before adding them to your routine for a really intense workout.

*A word of caution:* You should be extremely proficient at all these exercises on flat ground before you try them out on the BOSU Balance Trainer. They're not easy!

# ONE-LEG SQUAT

*This is the ultimate in strength, balance and coordination. If you can do this you're truly strong and fit. If necessary, use a table or chair to hold onto as you build your strength. Wearing a weighted vest intensifies the work.*

**STARTING POSITION:** Stand with both feet directly on either side of the bull's-eye. Find a stable position and engage your core.

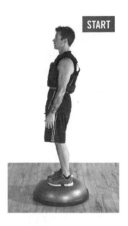

START

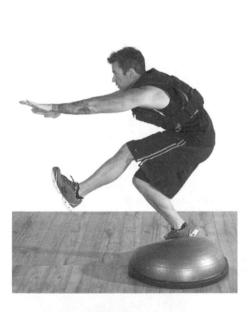

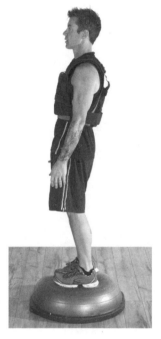

**1** Keeping your knee over your toe, bend your right knee and lower your body until your glutes drop as close as possible to parallel. Do not lean forward. Pause.

**2** Push up with your right leg, returning to starting position.

## VARIATION

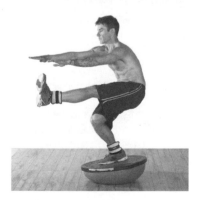

### NOTES

*Take care to notice differences in your legs. One leg is often stronger than the other, which means you need to work the weaker leg harder.*

*This movement alone could easily be considered a complete workout. One rotation contains 12 plyometric push-ups, and the stabilization required to keep your body flat while your toes are on the dome will really work your core and glutes. Your goal is to keep your toes on top of the dome with hands on the floor and perform push-ups while rotating clockwise or counter-clockwise in 12 different positions around the BOSU Balance Trainer. It sounds easier than it actually is. What? It doesn't sound easy? OK, we're on the same page then.*

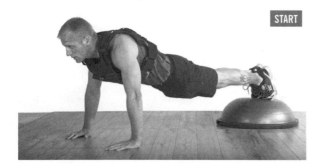

START

**STARTING POSITION:** Assume a push-up position with your toes on top of the dome—place your toes on the bull's-eye and both hands shoulder-width apart on the floor, arms fully extended. Keep your back flat and tighten your core to support your whole body.

**1** Bend both elbows and lower your body until your chest is 1–3 inches away from the floor. Pause.

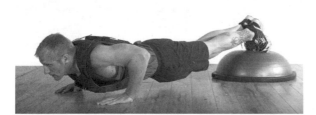

**2** Explode up, maintaining a straight back and legs while pushing yourself up and to the right (clockwise, left for counterclockwise rotation), back toward the top position. You need to use enough force to cause your hands to leave the ground. Everything should be off the floor; your toes remain on the dome.

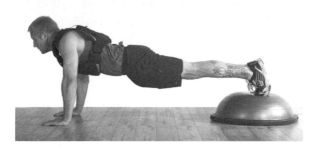

**3** Keeping your elbows slightly bent, softly land with both hands on the floor under your shoulders. With your toes remaining in place and rotating along with your body, continue working your way around in a circle. Go as far as you can before losing your form. Rest for 1 minute and try to return back to starting position by moving counterclockwise.

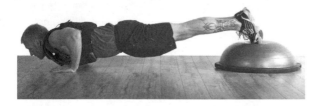

## NOTES

*Cushion the landing in your arms and shoulders. If you're too rigid, you're sure to get hurt. This is also a ridiculously effective core exercise, especially the way it requires keeping your hips square to maintain your toe placement on the apex of the dome.*

**START**

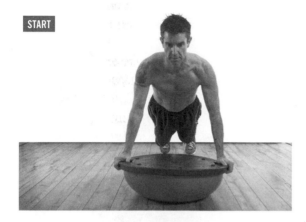

*If you enjoyed the Bounce-Ups and Around the Clock, you should be thrilled with this variation. Rotating either clockwise or counterclockwise and landing on the dome will activate just about every muscle from your fingertips to your toes in order to maintain your balance and keep your body in the proper position.*

**STARTING POSITION:** Get on your knees and grasp the sides of the flat surface, arms fully extended. Lift your knees off the floor and tighten your core to support your whole body.

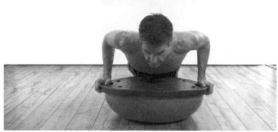

**1** Bend both elbows and lower your body until your chest touches the surface. Pause.

**2** Maintaining a straight back and legs, explode up while pushing yourself up and to the right (clockwise, left for counterclockwise rotation), back toward the plank position. You need to use enough force to cause your hands, still attached to the BOSU Balance Trainer, to leave the ground. Everything should be off the floor except for your toes.

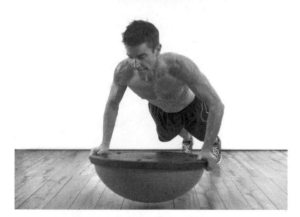

**3** Brace yourself and land with your elbows slightly bent. Lower your body until your chest touches the BOSU Balance Trainer. With your toes remaining in place and rotating along with your body, continue to work your way around in a circle.

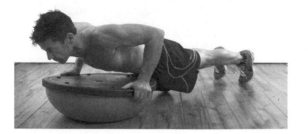

**NOTES**

*Cushion the landing in your arms and shoulders. If you're too rigid, you're sure to get hurt. This exercise is a series of explosive movements that's sure to work your body from head to toe.*

*Weren't burpees fun? Great! Glad you enjoyed them. This burpee variant is sure to have you sweating and swearing in a few reps. Wearing a weighted vest intensifies the work.*

**STARTING POSITION:** Stand approximately half a body's length behind the BOSU Balance Trainer.

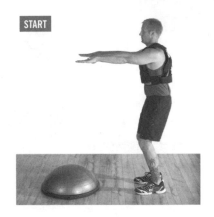

START

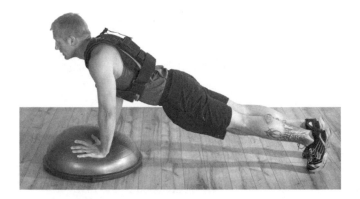

**1** Smoothly jump your feet backward and land softly on your toes. Simultaneously drop your upper body toward the BOSU Balance Trainer, softly landing your hands on either side of the bull's-eye.

**2** Bend your elbows and perform a push-up by lowering your chest to touch the top of the dome.

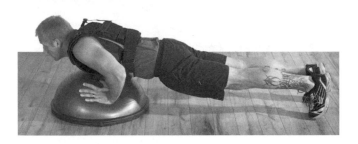

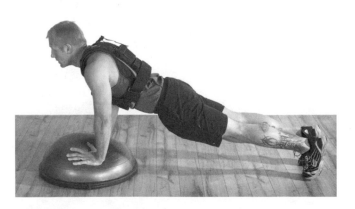

**3** Keeping your core engaged and back straight, use your chest and arms to raise your upper body into a plank position.

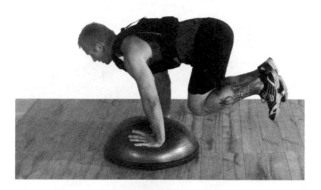

**4—5** Push upward off the dome with your arms while bending at the waist and jump your feet all the way to the BOSU Balance Trainer, landing softly on either side of the bull's-eye. You'll now be in a squat position with both feet on the dome of the BOSU Balance Trainer. Pushing through your heels, use your quads, hamstrings and glutes to raise your body up to a standing position.

That's 1 rep. Now carefully hop (or step) backward to starting position and repeat

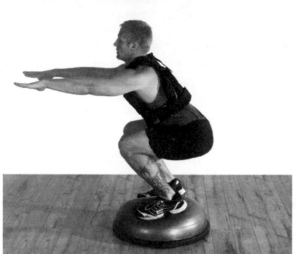

# TILT PLANK

*This is a core-shredding exercise all unto itself. The entire goal is to hold a plank as long as you can while rotating your hands into position to press the north, south, east and west edges of the BOSU Balance Trainer as close to the ground as possible.*

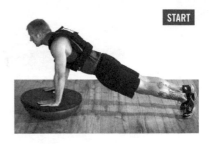

START

**STARTING POSITION:** Get on your knees and place your hands 2–3 inches apart in the center of the flat surface. Raise your knees off the ground, extend your legs fully and place your toes on the ground. Engage your core to straighten and support your back. Your body should form a straight line from head to heels.

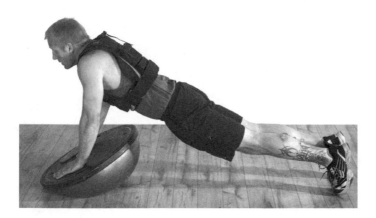

**1** Walk your hands out in front of you as far as you can, pressing the edge of the BOSU Balance Trainer toward the floor. Pause for as long as you can hold it.

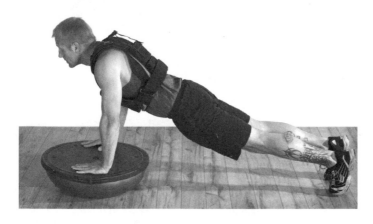

**2** Walk your hands back to the center. Rest as needed on your knees between position changes.

**3** Walk your hands as far to the right as you can. Pause, then return your hands to center.

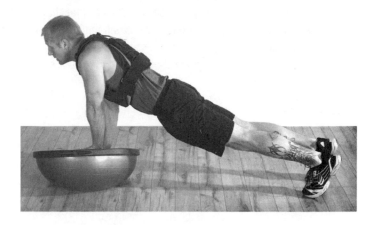

**4** Walk your hands as far to the left as you can. Pause, then return your hands to center.

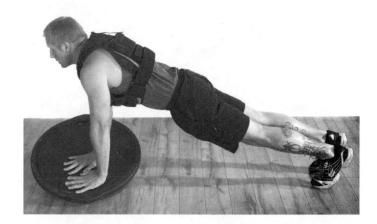

**5** Walk your hands as close as possible to the rim closest to your belly. Pause, then return your hands to center. That's 1 rep.

Rest and repeat.

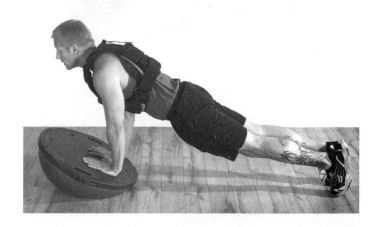

# BURPEE WITH OVERHEAD PRESS & LUNGE

*Hey, wait...where are the weights? Did you forget that the BOSU Balance Trainer weighs in around 13 pounds and has handles that are perfect for overhead presses? Well, here's your excuse to use one to perform an exercise that will work your entire body and surely turn some heads in the gym.*

**STARTING POSITION:** Stand approximately half a body's length behind the BOSU Balance Trainer, dome-side down.

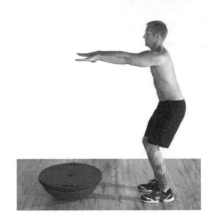

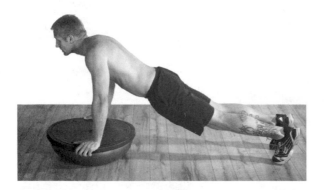

**1** Smoothly jump your feet backward, landing softly on your toes. Simultaneously drop your upper body toward the BOSU Balance Trainer, softly landing your hands on the outside rim of the flat base, and grab the handles.

**2** Keeping your core tight and back flat, perform a push-up by slowly lowering your chest to touch the flat side.

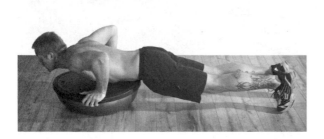

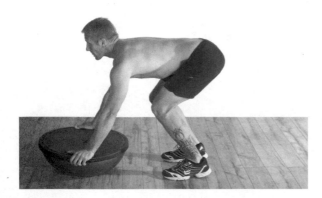

**3** Still gripping the handles, use your arms and chest to explosively push your upper body away from the BOSU Balance Trainer while bending at the waist and jumping your feet forward, back under your body. Land with your knees bent in a semi-squatting position (approximately 45 degrees).

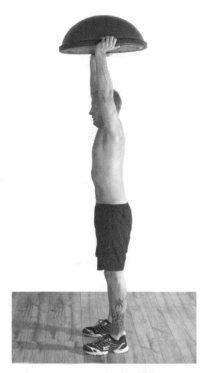

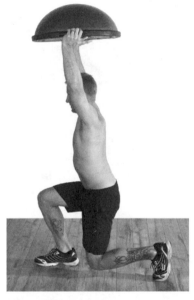

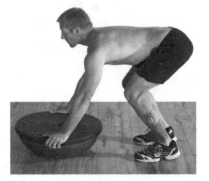

**4** Stand up straight, lifting the BOSU Balance Trainer and pressing it directly above your head.

**5** Step forward with your right foot and lower your left knee straight down in a lunge (see page 76); stop when both knees are bent 90 degrees. Keep your back straight and arms fully extended.

**6** Press off your right foot and left toes to return to standing, squat and lower the BOSU Balance Trainer back to the floor. That's 1 rep. Repeat with other leg.

**NOTES**

*C'mon, you have to admit that this was a pretty fun exercise! Tough, yes, but surely fun at the same time. Who knew that the BOSU Balance Trainer is effective as a weight too!*

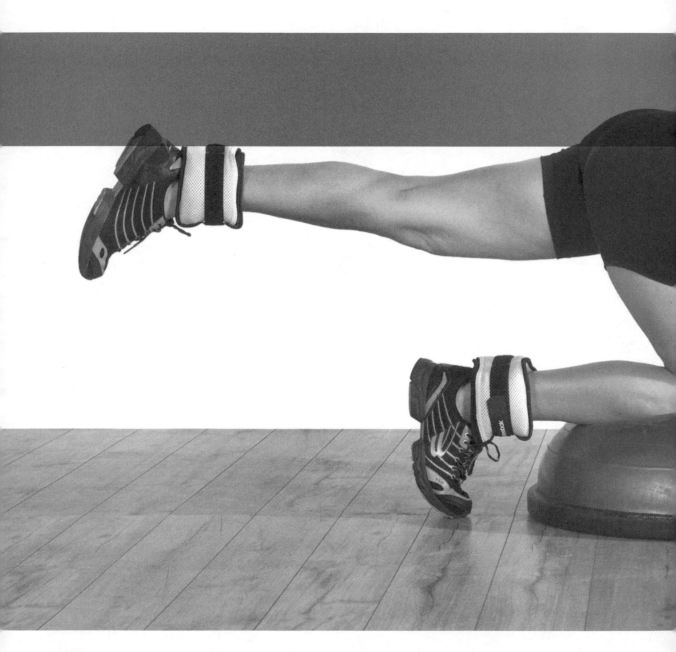

# PART 4

# APPENDIX

# Warm-Ups

As we discussed in "Preparing for the Workouts" on page 37, since you'll be pushing, pressing and lifting your bodyweight or additional weights on an unstable surface, it's very important to warm up before you work out or stretch. Stretching prior to warming up can cause more damage than good to muscles, ligaments and joints. When your muscles are cold, they're far less pliable and you don't receive any benefit from stretching prior to warming up. Below are some dynamic warm-ups that'll get your heart rate up, loosen tight muscles and prepare you for your workout.

# ARM CIRCLE

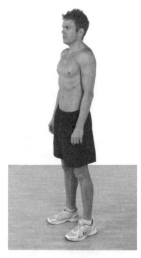 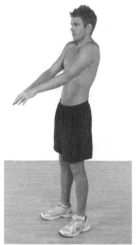

**1** Stand with your feet shoulder-width apart.

**2–3** Move both arms in a complete circle forward 5 times and then backward 5 times.

# LUMBER JACK

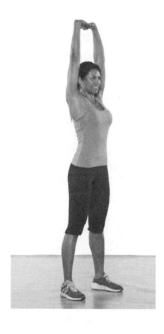 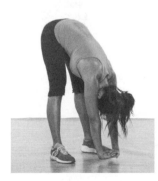

**1** Stand with your feet shoulder-width apart and extend your hands overhead with elbows locked, fingers interlocked and palms up.

**2** Bend forward at the waist and try to put your hands on the ground (like you're chopping wood).

Raise up and repeat.

# SIDE BEND

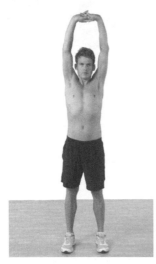

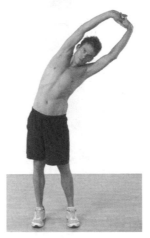 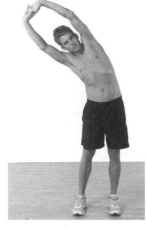

**1** Stand with your feet shoulder-width apart and extend your hands overhead with elbows locked, fingers interlocked and palms up.

**2–3** Bend side to side.

# AROUND THE WORLD

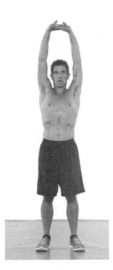

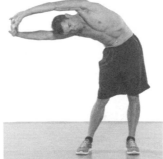 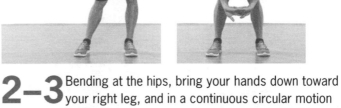

**1** Stand with your feet shoulder-width apart and extend your hands overhead with elbows locked, fingers interlocked and palms up. Keep your arms straight the entire time.

**2–3** Bending at the hips, bring your hands down toward your right leg, and in a continuous circular motion bring your hands toward your toes, then toward your left leg and then return your hands overhead and bend backward.

Repeat three times, then change directions.

# BARN DOORS

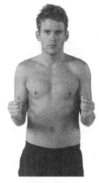 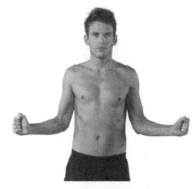

**1** Stand with your feet shoulder-width apart with your arms tight against your sides. Bend your arms 90 degrees so that your forearms extend forward and are parallel to the floor. Grip your hands like you have a rubber band between them.

**2** Keeping your forearms parallel to the floor, squeeze your shoulder blades together and pull your hands apart to the sides.

Do 10–12 reps.

# CHEST FLY

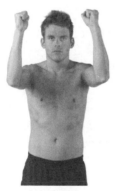 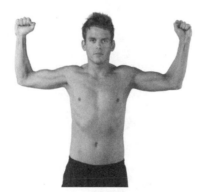

**1** Assume the Barn Doors position (above) with your hands in front of your torso, then raise your hands and elbows straight up, maintaining the 90-degree angle until your elbows are at shoulder height.

**2** Squeezing your shoulder blades together, pull your hands away from each other until your hands are parallel to your ears.

Do 10–12 reps.

# MARCHING TWIST

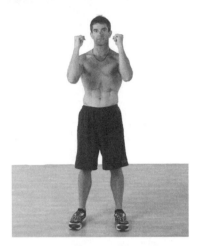

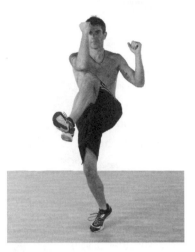

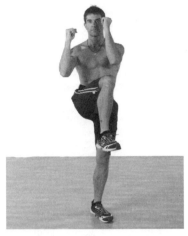

**1** Stand tall with your feet shoulder-width apart. Bring your arms in front of you and bend your elbows 90 degrees.

**2** Twist your torso to the right and raise your left knee to your right elbow.

**3** Repeat with your right knee and left elbow. A little hop with the bottom foot helps you keep your momentum going from leg to leg.

Do 10 reps on each leg.

# JUMPING JACKS

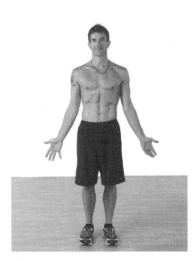

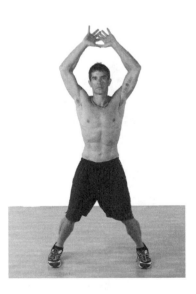

**2** Jump 6–12 inches off the ground and simultaneously spread your feet apart an additional 20–30 inches while extending your hands directly overhead.

Jump 6–12 inches off the ground and return your hands and feet to the starting position. Do 10 reps.

**1** Stand tall with your feet together and arms extended along your sides, palms facing forward.

# Stretches

After your workout, stretching will help you reduce soreness, increase range of motion and flexibility within a joint or muscle, and prepare your body for any future workouts. Stretching immediately after exercise while your muscles are still warm allows your muscles to return to their full range of motion (which gives you more flexibility gains) and reduces the chance of injury or fatigue in the hours or days after an intense workout.

It's important to remember that even when you're warm and loose, you should never "bounce" during stretching. Keep your movements slow and controlled. The stretches in this section should be performed in order to optimize your recovery. Remember to exhale as you perform every deep stretch and rest 30 seconds in between each stretch.

# FOREARM & WRIST

*Begin the stretch gently and allow your forearms to relax before stretching them to their full range of motion.*

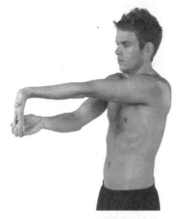

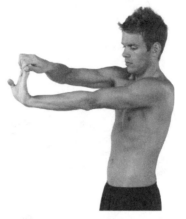

**1** Stand with your feet shoulder-width apart and extend both arms straight out in front of you. Keep your back straight. Turn your left wrist to the sky and grasp your left fingers from below with your right hand. Slowly pull your fingers back toward your torso with your right hand. Hold for 10 seconds. Swap arms and repeat.

**2** Now perform the stretch with your fingers pointing up.

# SHOULDERS

**1** Stand with your feet shoulder-width apart and bring your left arm across your chest. Support your left elbow with the crook of your right arm by raising your right arm to 90 degrees. Gently pull your left arm to your chest while maintaining proper posture (straight back, wide shoulders). Don't round or hunch your shoulders. Hold your arm to your chest for 10 seconds.

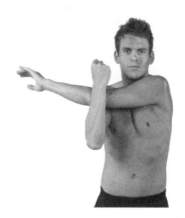

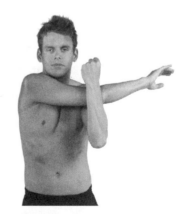

**2** Release and switch arms.

After you've done both sides, shake your hands out for 5–10 seconds.

# SHOULDERS & UPPER BACK

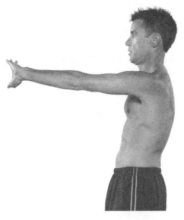 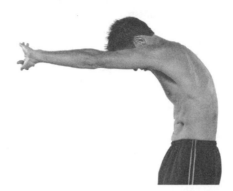

**1** Stand with your feet shoulder-width apart and extend both arms straight out in front of you. Interlace your fingers and turn your palms to face away from your body. Keep your back straight.

**2** Reach your palms away from your body. Exhale as you push your palms straight out from your body by pushing through your shoulders and upper back. Allow your neck to bend naturally as you round your upper back. Continue to reach your hands and stretch for 10 seconds.

Rest for 30 seconds then repeat. After you've done the second set, shake your arms out for 10 seconds to your sides to return blood to the fingers and forearm muscles.

## CHEST

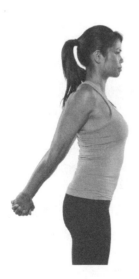

**1** Clasp your hands together behind your lower back with palms facing each other. Keeping an erect posture and your arms as straight as possible, gently pull your arms away from your back, straight out behind you. Keep your shoulders down. Hold for 10 seconds.

Rest for 30 seconds and repeat.

# ARMS

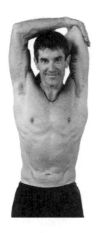

**1** Stand with your feet shoulder-width apart. Maintaining a straight back, grab your elbows with the opposite hand. Slowly raise your arms until they're slightly behind your head. Keeping your right hand on your left elbow, drop your left hand to the top of your right shoulder blade. Gently push your left elbow down with your right hand, and hold for 10 seconds.

Rest for 10 seconds and then repeat with opposite arms.

# LOWER BACK

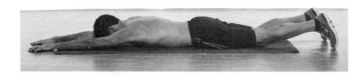

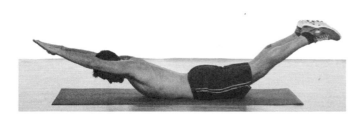

**1** Lying face-down on your stomach, extend your arms along the floor above your head, palms on the ground. Keeping your knees straight, extend your legs behind you, keeping your feet close together and your toes on the ground.

**2** In a slow, controlled motion, contract your lower back (erector spinae) and raise your arms and legs 6–8 inches off the floor. Hold for 5 seconds.

Lower slowly back to starting position. Repeat slowly 10 times.

# NECK

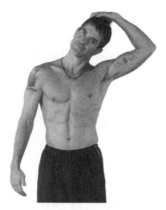 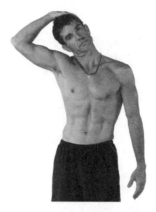

**1** Standing like a soldier (with your back straight, shoulders square and chest raised), slowly lower your left ear to your left shoulder. To increase the stretch, use your left hand to gently pull your head toward your shoulder. Hold for 5–10 seconds.

**2** Slowly roll your chin to your chest and then lower your right ear to your right shoulder, again using your hand to enhance the stretch. Hold for 5–10 seconds.

Return your head to normal position and then tilt back slightly and look straight up. Hold for 5–10 seconds.

# Index

# Acknowledgments

Thanks to our friends and family for their support and willingness to give us the benefit of the doubt when we ask, "What if we try this?" Nearly all of our workout programs have started with these five little words.

The tenacity award goes to Brian and Tricia Burns for soldiering through multiple photo shoots despite Brian's broken foot and Tricia's pregnancy. You guys are truly great friends and amazing athletes.

Thanks to Brian Peitz of Fuzion Fitness in Scottsdale and Glendale, Arizona, for providing equipment and support.

Most importantly, thanks to our newest model Kristen for making us both very proud!

# About the Authors

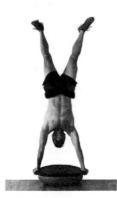

*Author Brett Stewart*

**Brett Stewart** is an endurance athlete and certified personal trainer residing in Phoenix, Arizona. An adrenaline junkie, Brett is an Ironman triathlete, ultra-marathoner and rabid obstacle racer. A proud father, husband, son and brother, Brett has written numerous fitness books including *7 Weeks to a Triathlon*, *7 Weeks to Getting Ripped*, *7 Weeks to 10 Pounds of Muscle* and *Ultimate Obstacle Race Training*.

**Jason Warner** is an ISSA Certified Strength Trainer, fitness and sports enthusiast, ultra-marathoner, triathlete, CrossFitter and overall Olympic-lifting nut. He recently relocated to Victoria, British Columbia, from Adelaide, South Australia, with his wife and two young children. Jason wrote *Ultimate Jump Rope Workouts* and *7 Weeks to 10 Pounds of Muscle*, and contributed heavily to *7 Weeks to 50 Pull-Ups* and *7 Weeks to Getting Ripped*.

Contact Jason and Brett and sample any of their fitness programs, books and mobile apps at 7weekstofitness.com.